Type 2 Diabetes in Childhood and Adolescence

A global perspective

Edited by

Martin Silink MD
Institute of Endocrinology & Diabetes
University of Sydney
The Children's Hospital at Westmead, Australia

Kaichi Kida MD PhD
Department of Paediatrics
Ehime University School of Medicine, Japan

Arlan L Rosenbloom MD
Department of Pediatrics
University of Florida College of Medicine
Gainesville, USA

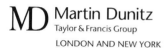

Martin Dunitz
Taylor & Francis Group
LONDON AND NEW YORK

© 2003 Martin Dunitz, an imprint of the Taylor & Francis Group plc

First published in the United Kingdom in 2003
by Martin Dunitz, an imprint of the Taylor & Francis Group plc, 11 New Fetter
Lane, London EC4P 4EE

Tel.: +44 (0) 20 7583 9855
Fax.: +44 (0) 20 7842 2298
E-mail: info@dunitz.co.uk
Website: http://www.dunitz.co.uk

A CIP record for this book is available from the British Library.

ISBN 1 84184 295 8

Distributed in the USA by
Fulfilment Center
Taylor & Francis
10650 Toebben Drive
Independence, KY 41051, USA
Toll Free Tel.: +1 800 634 7064
E-mail: taylorandfrancis@thomsonlearning.com

Distributed in Canada by
Taylor & Francis
74 Rolark Drive
Scarborough, Ontario M1R 4G2, Canada
Toll Free Tel.: +1 877 226 2237
E-mail: tal_fran@istar.ca

Distributed in the rest of the world by
Thomson Publishing Services
Cheriton House
North Way
Andover, Hampshire SP10 5BE, UK
Tel.: +44 (0)1264 332424
E-mail: salesorder.tandf@thomsonpublishingservices.co.uk

Printed and bound in Great Britain by The Cromwell Press Ltd, Trowbridge

Contents

Contributors

Silva A Arslanian MD
University of Pittsburgh, Children's Hospital of Pittsburgh, 3705 Fifth Avenue, Pittsburgh, PA 15213, USA

Louise A Baur MB BS BSc(Med) PhD
University of Sydney, Discipline of Paediatrics & Child Health, The Children's Hospital at Westmead, Locked Bag 4001, Westmead NSW 2145, Australia

Paul Czernichow MD
INSERM Unité 457, Hôpital Robert Debré, 75019 Paris, France

Denis Daneman MD
Department of Pediatrics, University of Toronto and The Hospital for Sick Children, Toronto, Canada M5G 1X8

Elizabeth Denney-Wilson BNurs MPH
University of Sydney, Discipline of Paediatrics & Child Health, The Children's Hospital at Westmead, Locked Bag 4001 Westmead NSW 2145, Australia

Jill Hamilton MD
Department of Pediatrics, University of Toronto and The Hospital for Sick Children, Toronto, Canada M5G 1X8

Giuseppina Imperatore MD PhD
Division of Diabetes Translation, National Center for Chronic Disease Prevention and Health Promotion, Centers for Disease Control and Prevention, 4770 Buford Highway, Atlanta, GA 30341, USA

Delphine Jaquet MD
INSERM Unité 457, Hôpital Robert Debré, 75019 Paris, France

Kenneth L Jones MD
Department of Pediatrics, University of California, San Diego, 9500 Gilman Drive, La Jolla, CA 92093, USA

Kaichi Kida MD PhD
Department of Paediatrics, Ehime University School of Medicine, Shitsukawa, Shigenobu, Ehime 791-0295, Japan

Claire Lévy-Marchal MD
INSERM Unité 457, Hôpital Robert Debré, 75019 Paris, France

Susan A Phillips MD
Department of Pediatrics, University of California, San Diego, 9500 Gilman Drive, La Jolla, CA 92093, USA

Arlan L Rosenbloom MD
Department of Pediatrics, University of Florida College of Medicine, Children's Medical Services Center, 1701 SW 16th Avenue, Building B, Gainesville, FL 32608, USA

Martin Silink MD
Institute of Endocrinology and Diabetes, University of Sydney, The Children's Hospital at Westmead, Locked Bag 4001, Westmead NSW 2145, Australia

Yasuko Uchigata MD
Diabetes Center, Tokyo Women's Medical, University School of Medicine, 8-1 Kawada-cho, Shinjuku-ku, Tokyo 162-8666, Japan

Frank Vinicor MD MPH
Division of Diabetes Translation, National Center for Chronic Disease Prevention and Health Promotion, Centers for Disease Control and Prevention, 4770 Buford Highway, Atlanta, GA 30341, USA

Desmond E Williams MB ChB PhD
Division of Diabetes Translation, National Center for Chronic Disease Prevention and Health Promotion, Centers for Disease Control and Prevention, 4770 Buford Highway, Atlanta, GA 30341, USA

William E Winter MD
Department of Pathology, Immunology & Laboratory Medicine, University of Florida, Box 100275, Gainesville, FL 32610, USA

Preface

Type 2 diabetes now affects over 5% of the world's population and is affecting progressively younger populations. This epidemic of type 2 diabetes parallels the global increase in obesity. The reasons for these concomitant epidemics remain poorly understood, but involve the complex interactions of genetic predisposition, prenatal environment, and the major lifestyle and environmental changes brought about by modernization, industrialization, and globalization.

Previously regarded as a disease of adults, type 2 diabetes is now seen in adolescence and even childhood. Pediatricians and physicians caring for the young have to decide whether a newly diagnosed child or adolescent with diabetes has type 1 diabetes, type 2 diabetes, ADM (atypical diabetes mellitus), MODY (maturity onset diabetes of the young), or one of the other recently described forms of diabetes. In some parts of the world, such as Japan, type 2 diabetes has become more prevalent than type 1 diabetes, even in childhood and adolescence.

This book provides a state-of-the-art review and is aimed at pediatricians, physicians, medical students, diabetes educators, and other medical health professionals involved in the care of children and adolescents with type 2 diabetes. In this volume, international experts address the interrelationship of diabetes, obesity, insulin resistance and the metabolic syndrome, the spectrum of clinical features and diagnostic issues, the epidemiology, pathophysiologic basis, genetics, and the treatment of type 2 diabetes in children and adolescents.

While there is a large body of information on type 2 diabetes in adults, there are relatively few data on this disease in childhood and adolescence. The available data in type 2 diabetes of young onset indicate that the microvascular complications of diabetes (retinopathy and nephropathy) are as severe and as frequent as in type 1 diabetes, while the macrovascular complications are greatly accelerated. Children and adolescents with type 2 diabetes will face the major complications of diabetes as young adults, unless effective therapy can prevent these.

The management of children and adolescents with type 2 diabetes is complex and involves the whole family and the resources of the community. The treatment may involve weight reduction, lifestyle modification, exercise programs, and medications to treat the hyperglycemia. Few of the drugs used in the treatment of type 2 diabetes and even fewer of those used to reduce the risk of cardiovascular disease have been licensed for use in childhood and adolescence.

The direct and indirect costs of diabetes and obesity are consuming a large proportion of health care resources in both developing and developed nations. Children and adolescents with diabetes face a lifetime of therapy and the likelihood of complications in young adulthood at a time when family commitments and productivity should be at their peak. The prevention of type 2 diabetes and obesity have become urgent issues for all age groups, but especially so for children and adolescents.

Martin Silink
Kaichi Kida
Arlan L Rosenbloom

chapter 1

Introduction – global evolution of diabetes in children and adolescents

Martin Silink, Kaichi Kida, and Arlan L Rosenbloom

Evolution is usually a process of slow change that can only be appreciated after a considerable amount of time has passed. Although we think of epidemics as being more revolutionary than evolutionary, we have witnessed the evolution of two concurrent global non-communicable disease epidemics, or pandemics, in less than 25 years. The epidemics of obesity and type 2 diabetes, unlike acute and time-limited epidemics of infections in the past, pose an insidious and continuing profound effect on individual and public health. These pandemics are intimately linked, with the epidemic of obesity preceding and setting the scene for the development of type 2 diabetes. In the evolutionary process, these diseases are now affecting progressively younger age groups. No longer can we think of type 2 diabetes as maturity onset diabetes. In many parts of the world and among certain ethnic groups, the incidence of type 2 diabetes in the adolescent age group is now equal to or greater than that of type 1 diabetes and it is even being recognized in prepubertal children, as young as 4–6 years in the USA and UK.[1]

Although 2–3% of pediatric diabetes had been recognized as being type 2 at least 30 years ago,[2-4] type 2 diabetes has only emerged as a common pediatric disease in the past decade.[5] Concomitantly, recognition of the epidemic of obesity and its multiple deleterious effects on lifelong health, of which type 2 diabetes is only one aspect, has moved this disease of civilization to the forefront of pediatric concerns.

Pediatricians need to deal with these challenging problems, and understand their etiology, their morbidity, and what possible treatments are available. Much remains unknown.

The global epidemic of type 2 diabetes parallels the increasing global prevalence of obesity. In the USA, obesity rates exceed 20% of the population. In the USA in 1988, data from the Centers for Disease Control and Prevention (CDC) revealed that only 19 states had a prevalence of obesity of 10–14% and none had a documented prevalence in excess of this. By 1995, 27 states had a prevalence of obesity of 15–19%, with the remainder having a prevalence of 10–14%. The situation continued to deteriorate and, by 2000, 23 states in the USA had a prevalence of obesity in excess of 20%, 26 with a prevalence of 15–19%, and only one with a prevalence of 10–14%.[6] These alarming data have been mirrored by similar rises in many other parts of the world. Children and adolescents have not been exempt and a prevalence of obesity in excess of 10% has been recorded from such disparate countries as Thailand, Japan, Australia, the USA, Italy, and the UK.

The documented increase in obesity in the USA has been accompanied by an equally well-documented rise in type 2 diabetes. In 1990, only four states had a prevalence of diabetes >6% but, by 2000, 20 states had a prevalence >6%.[7]

The World Health Organization (WHO) has calculated that in 1995 there were approximately 130 million people with type 2 diabetes globally. These figures increased to 150 million in 2000, 172 million in 2002, and the projection is for there to be 300 million people with diabetes by 2025. Currently, there are no figures for type 2 diabetes in adolescents and children.

The relationship between obesity and disordered glucose regulation has also been demonstrated in childhood and adolescence. A recent study from Yale University demonstrated that of 55 obese children aged 4–10 years 25% had impaired glucose tolerance (IGT). In obese adolescents aged 11–18 years, 21% had IGT and a further 4% had previously undiagnosed type 2 diabetes.[8]

The link between a sedentary lifestyle with obesity and the development of diabetes is through insulin resistance. Obesity and inactivity both reduce insulin sensitivity and therefore require the pancreatic beta cells to secrete increased amounts of insulin. Progressive beta-cell failure results in impaired insulin secretion and the consequent loss of glucose regulation. Chronic hyperglycemia is thought to induce beta-cell apoptosis, irreversible insulin deficiency, and permanent diabetes. The progression of the metabolic abnormalities from normal glycemic homeostasis to type 2 diabetes has several intermediate stages which can be detected as impaired fasting glycemia (IFG) or as IGT (Figure 1.1). Genetic variations in insulin resistance have been documented among various ethnic groups and may contribute to the increased susceptibility to diabetes in these populations (the thrifty genotype hypothesis). Intrauterine environmental factors may also influence lifelong insulin sensitivity and beta-cell function (the thrifty phenotype hypothesis).[9]

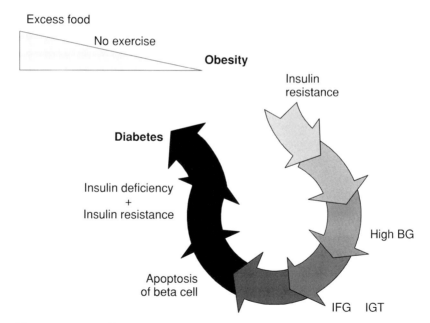

Figure 1.1 *The effects of excess calories and a sedentary lifestyle in leading to the development of obesity, insulin resistance, impaired glucose homeostasis and, finally, type 2 diabetes. BG = blood glucose; IFG = impaired fasting glucose, IGT = impaired glucose tolerance.*

In many countries, the increase in type 2 diabetes has occurred with a concurrent well-documented increase in immune-mediated diabetes (type 1 diabetes). Although these two forms of diabetes seem quite distinct, the accelerator hypothesis suggests that beta-cell damage from chronic hyperglycemia may induce release of beta-cell immunogens.[10]

The worldwide increases in obesity rates are due to people consuming more energy than they expend. For the average person a net accumulation of 1% of daily food energy will result in a 1 kg weight gain over a year. This net excess in caloric intake can result from eating this amount more each day or expending fewer calories in exercise. This simple formulation does not reflect the complexity of the situation. The causes of obesity involve psychosocial factors as well as the simple acts of over-eating or under-exercising. Studies have shown that people tend to consume a similar bulk of food each day. Eating the same bulk of more energy-dense food will inevitably increase caloric intake.[11]

Despite famine and starvation affecting about 800 million of the world's population, the fact remains that, for the remainder, never in the history of man has so much food been so readily available to so many. The previous feast–famine cycles have been replaced by more or less continuous feasting. Foods are increasingly made calorie dense with high fat content and with highly refined carbohydrate, and often have low satiation value. Flavor enhancers help to promote appetite. Even the texture of food is designed to appeal to the palate and its presentation is visually attractive. Give away toys with foods determine choice and portion size has become larger – 'value for money'.

Drinks are increasingly high in calories as the shift is to bottled or canned drinks. Thirst is thus being slaked not with water but with sweet energy-containing drinks that further stimulate appetite and thirst. Drink volumes are being determined by the size of the can or bottle rather than by the magnitude of thirst.

With the urbanization of societies, exercise is no longer part of every-day life. School curricula do not include exercise as such and there has been an emphasis on sport and winning versus exercising for health. Television, videos, and computers have all contributed to more time being spent on sedentary activities. Exercise not only consumes energy but also increases insulin sensitivity, predominantly by increasing glucose flux through the GLUT4 transporters present in insulin-sensitive tissues such as skeletal muscle. Moderate activity of 30 min/day has been shown to improve insulin sensitivity. However, sedentary lifestyles are the norm.

The 20th century witnessed a major population increase, the progressive urbanization of societies, and the formation of mega-cities. Major lifestyle changes have occurred in accommodating to this new environment, which is often hostile and filled with traffic. The place of employment for people is increasingly distant from home, making use of public or private transport a necessity. Similarly, children need to be driven to schools or have to use public transport. Homework, academic pursuits, and work competition contribute to long hours in sedentary circumstances. Playgrounds have disappeared in many areas and have been transformed into sterile manicured parks in others. Neighborhoods may not be safe for children to play outside.

Family issues contribute to the increasing move to prepackaged high-energy foods and decreased exercise. In many societies, there has been disintegration of the extended family along with divorce rates of 40–50%. Children have to cope with both parents at work or being part of single-parent families. Many families simply do not have the time to prepare food or may have lost the skills to be able to prepare it. Prepackaged or fast foods offer easy alternatives but suffer the disadvantage of being high in fat and energy.

Societal perceptions of obesity are also changing. Mothers tend to be aware of their own overweight or obese state but not that of their children.[12]

The importance of stress as part of modern lifestyles in the genesis of obesity and diabetes is gaining acceptance. Coronary vascular risk was doubled in white-collar workers who felt they had low control over their jobs and who perceived little reward for the effort expended in their work.[13] Elegant studies in animal models as well as human studies indicate a role of the hypothalamo–pituitary–adrenal axis in the pathogenesis of the metabolic syndrome.[14]

The treatment of type 2 diabetes in childhood and adolescence is especially difficult. Internationally, the only drugs licensed for use in the treatment of type 2 diabetes in childhood and adolescence are insulin itself and metformin, with metformin being the drug of choice for those able to be weaned off insulin or those whose hyperglycemia is not too severe. Other drugs, while available and effective, are used 'off-licence'.

Type 2 diabetes causes both macro- and microvascular complications of diabetes. The mechanism of this damaging process is slowly becoming understood and involves oxidative and glycation processes. It is fascinating to consider that glucose and oxygen are sustainers of life yet both are major determinants of the damaging aging processes. Both lead to tissue damage directly and indirectly: oxygen, through production of reactive oxygen species; glucose, through glycation of proteins. Evidence now indicates that type 2 diabetes is just as capable as type 1 diabetes of causing serious morbidity and increased mortality. Children and adolescents with type 2 diabetes thus face these complications in early adulthood. The lessons learned from the UKPDS (United Kingdom Prospective Diabetes Study) that intensified treatment reduces the risk of complications need to be applied to the treatment of type 2 diabetes in the young and this requires close follow-up.

Recognizing the difficulties of treatment of type 2 diabetes, the long-term aim should be primary prevention. Primary prevention of disorders of glucose homeostasis will need to focus on reducing insulin resistance to which obesity and a sedentary lifestyle are the most important contributors. The global epidemic of obesity and diabetes will not be reversed until the environmental and lifestyle issues are addressed effectively. There is now incontrovertible proof that lifestyle modification (modest weight reduction and daily exercise equivalent to 30 min of brisk walking) significantly decreases the risk of patients with IGT progressing to diabetes.[15,16]

The solutions are public health and societal ones. Examples of healthy practices, which still need the fullness of time to demonstrate their effectiveness, include the National School Fruit Program in the UK. Singapore has 12 years' experience with the TAF Program (trim and fit) in which all schools have to publish the prevalence of obesity, overweight, and fitness ranking in their school. Incentives are provided to the school for improvements in these parameters. Education on eating and lifestyle changes for the whole family are part of this program. Preliminary data indicate that the increase in obesity in schoolchildren has largely been contained.

The food and drink industry needs to produce less energy-dense foods, but will only do so if the market demands it. Data from Wisconsin show the positive effect of price reduction on the sales of low-fat snacks, whereas health promotion education had little impact. Television advertising of snack foods aimed at school-age children needs to be limited, especially during their peak viewing times, but whether this is achieved by industry-led codes of practice or government regulation is being debated.

The recent filing of class-action lawsuits against certain fast-food chains in the USA, citing the addictive nature of fast foods and the lack of health warnings on fast foods containing high fat, is being watched with interest. Perhaps the fear of litigation may lead to changes towards healthier fast foods. The banning of soft drink and snack machines from schools in several county school districts in the USA is an important beginning.

What is clear is that the problem of obesity and diabetes is very great. Preventive action is urgently needed and will require a broad societal initiative. The time for inaction and complacency is past.

References

1. Ehtisham S, Barrett TG, Shaw NJ. Type 2 diabetes mellitus in UK children – an emerging problem. *Diabetic Med* 2000; **17**(12):867–71.
2. Knowles HC. Diabetes mellitus in childhood and adolescence. *Med Clin N Am* 1971; **55**:975–87.
3. Drash AM. Relationship between diabetes mellitus and obesity in the child. *Metabolism* 1973; **22**:337–44.
4. Martin MM, Martin AL. Obesity, hyperinsulinism, and diabetes mellitus in childhood. *J Pediatr* 1973; **82**(2):92–201.
5. Rosenbloom AL, Joe JR, Young RS, Winter WE. Emerging epidemic of type 2 diabetes in youth. *Diabetes Care* 1999; **22**(2):345–54.
6. Mokdad AH, Bowman BA, Ford ES, Vinicor F, Marks JS, Koplan JP. The continuing epidemics of obesity and diabetes in the United States. *JAMA* 2001; **286**(10):1195–200.
7. Mokdad AH, Ford ES, Bowman BA *et al*. Diabetes trends in the U.S.: 1990–1998. *Diabetes Care* 2000; **23**(9):1278–83.
8. Sinha R, Fisch G, Teague B *et al*. Prevalence of impaired glucose tolerance among children and adolescents with marked obesity. *N Engl J Med* 2002; **346**(11):802–10.

9. Hales CN, Barker DJ. Type 2 (non-insulin-dependent) diabetes mellitus: the thrifty phenotype hypothesis. *Diabetologia* 1992; **35**(7):595–601.
10. Wilkin TJ. The accelerator hypothesis: weight gain as the missing link between type I and type II diabetes. *Diabetologia* 2001; **44**(7):914–22.
11. Prentice AM. Manipulation of dietary fat and energy density and subsequent effects on substrate flux and food intake. *Am J Clin Nutr* 1998; **67**(3 suppl): 535–41S.
12. Baughcum AE, Chamberlin LA, Deeks CM, Powers SW, Whitaker RC. Maternal perceptions of overweight preschool children. *Pediatrics* 2000; **106**(6):1380–6.
13. Bosma H, Peter R, Siegrist J, Marmot M. Two alternative job stress models and the risk of coronary heart disease. *Am J Publ Health* 1998; **88**(1):68–74.
14. Bjorntorp P, Rosmond R. The metabolic syndrome – a neuroendocrine disorder? *Br J Nutr* 2000; **83**(suppl 1):S49–57.
15. Tuomilehto J, Lindstrom J, Eriksson JG *et al.* Prevention of type 2 diabetes mellitus by changes in lifestyle among subjects with impaired glucose tolerance. *N Engl J Med* 2001; **344**(18):1343–50.
16. Pan XR, Li GW, Hu YH *et al.* Effects of diet and exercise in preventing NIDDM with impaired glucose tolerance. The Da Qing IGT and Diabetes Study. *Diabetes Care* 1997; **20**(4):537–44.

chapter 2

Diagnosis and classification of type 2 diabetes in childhood and adolescence

Arlan L Rosenbloom and Martin Silink

Diagnosis

The diagnosis of diabetes mellitus encompasses a wide array of metabolic diseases characterized by chronic hyperglycemia. Because insulin is the only physiologically significant hypoglycemic hormone, hyperglycemia must be the result of either impaired insulin secretion by the beta cells of the pancreas, resistance to the effect of insulin in the liver, muscle, and fat cells, or a combination of these pathophysiologic situations. It is important to recognize that the hyperglycemia of diabetes is not simply a reflection of abnormal glucose metabolism, but the result of disturbed energy metabolism from inadequate insulin action with widespread disturbances in carbohydrate, fat, and protein metabolism.

Criteria for the diagnosis of diabetes were revised several years ago by the American Diabetes Association (ADA) and the World Health Organization (WHO).[1,2] The major change in the revised criteria for the diagnosis of diabetes has been a lowering of the diagnostic level of fasting plasma glucose from $\geq$7.8 mmol/l (140 mg%) to $\leq$7.0 mmol/l (126 mg%).

Also in the revised criteria, categories of impaired fasting glucose (IFG) and impaired glucose tolerance (IGT) were added because of recognition that these abnormalities are associated with increased cardiovascular morbidity, and the ADA has recommended that IFG and IGT be

regarded as constituting a state of prediabetes. These terms are not inter-
changeable, representing different abnormalities or stages of abnormality in glucose regulation. IFG is an abnormality of glucose homeostasis
in the fasting state whereas IGT can only be diagnosed by a 2-h post-
load reading following a standard oral glucose intake. Long-term studies
in children and adolescents are not yet available, but longitudinal data
in adults indicate that after 5–10 years, those with IGT have similar poss-
ibilities of progressing to diabetes, reverting to normal, or remaining
with IGT (Figure 2.1).[3] Those with IFG have a 45% chance of reverting to
normal or remaining with IFG and approx 10% risk of progressing to
diabetes. Even though glucose homeostasis differs at various age and
developmental stages, circulating glucose levels do not significantly vary
with age (except at the extremes of age); thus, the ADA and WHO criteria for diagnosis of diabetes and prediabetes in childhood are the same
as for adults (Table 2.1).

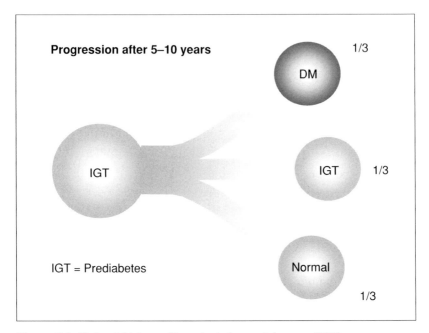

Figure 2.1 *Natural history of impaired glucose tolerance (IGT).*

Table 2.1 Criteria for the diagnosis of diabetes

✓ Symptoms plus
   random plasma glucose concentration ≥11.1 mmol/l (200 mg/dl),
✓ or fasting plasma glucose ≥7.0 mmol/l (126 mg/dl),
✓ or 2-h plasma glucose ≥11.1 mmol/l (200 mg/dl) during an oral glucose
   tolerance test (OGTT).

*The test should be performed in the morning, after an overnight fast of
8–14 h, using a glucose load containing the equivalent of 1.75 g/kg
anhydrous glucose up to a maximum of 75 g (i.e., 1.75 g/kg for those weighing
<43 kg and 75 g for those weighing > 43 kg). The glucose load should be
dissolved in 250–300 ml water and drunk over the course of 5 min. The test is
timed from the beginning of the drink. Before the OGTT, there should have been
at least 3 days of an unrestricted diet containing at least 150 g of carbohydrate
daily.*

Prediabetes:
   Impaired glucose tolerance (IGT) = 2-h plasma glucose ≥7.8 to
   <11.1 mmol/l (≥140 to <200 mg/dl)
   Impaired fasting glucose (IFG) = ≥ 6.1 to < 7.0 mmol/l (≥110 to
   <126 mg/dl)

In the absence of marked hyperglycemia with metabolic decompensation, abnormal values should be confirmed by repeat testing on a different day. The oral glucose tolerance test (OGTT) is not recommended for routine clinical use.[1] The WHO recommends that, 'for clinical purposes, an OGTT to establish diagnostic status need only be considered if casual blood glucose values lie in the uncertain range and the fasting blood glucoses are below those which establish the diagnosis of diabetes'.[2]

Classification

The classification of diabetes has been revised from that based on treatment to a largely etiologic taxonomy reflecting contemporary understanding of the pathogenesis of various forms of diabetes (e.g., type 1 diabetes instead of insulin-dependent diabetes mellitus or IDDM; type

Table 2.2 Classification of diabetes in children

- *Type 1*[a] (beta-cell destruction, usually leading to absolute insulin deficiency)
    1a. immune-mediated
    1b. idiopathic.
- *Type 2*[a] (may range from predominantly insulin resistance with relative insulin deficiency to a predominantly secretory defect with insulin resistance).
- *Other specific types* (e.g., genetic defects of beta-cell function or insulin action, cystic fibrosis, glucocorticoid induced, or with genetic syndromes).

[a] Patients with any form of diabetes may require insulin treatment at some stage of their disease. Use of insulin does not, of itself, classify the patient.

2 diabetes instead of non-insulin-dependent diabetes mellitus or NIDDM; other types of diabetes). An abbreviated classification is given in Table 2.2.

Although most patients can be readily classified as having type 1 or type 2 diabetes, there are a number of patients in whom the distinction is difficult to make and who share features of both type 1 and type 2 diabetes.

Type 1 diabetes

Type 1 diabetes, immune-mediated, occurs throughout childhood with similar peaks of incidence at about 7 and 12–13 years of age. It is much less frequent in Asians and native North Americans, and somewhat less frequent in African-Americans than in those of European origin. Only about 5–10% of newly diagnosed patients have affected first-degree relatives and there is an equal sex ratio. The disease is associated with human leukocyte antigen complex (HLA) specificities (which vary in different ethnic populations) and diabetes specific autoimmunity, indicated by the presence of circulating autoantibodies to insulin (IAA), islet cell cytoplasm (ICA), glutamic acid dehydrogenase (GAD), or tyrosine phosphatase (IA-2) in 85–98% of patients. Onset is typically associated with weight loss, polyuria, polydipsia, fatigue, and weakness; in infants and toddlers, non-specific symptoms are often not recognized as indicative of diabetes. Ketoacidosis may occur in as many as 40% of newly diagnosed patients in some settings. Insulin secretion, as demonstrated by C-peptide concentration, is very low or absent, although there may be a period of partial recovery following initial diagnosis and treatment that can last for months to (rarely) years.

Type 1 diabetes, idiopathic, may be difficult to differentiate from immune-mediated type 1 diabetes. This classification includes a variety of causes and these may be specific to different parts of the world and ethnic backgrounds. In Southeast Asian countries, up to 60% of young people with a clinical picture of type 1 diabetes (short duration of typical symptoms, non-obese, ketosis prone, insulin-deficient, and total dependence on insulin) may not have GAD autoantibodies which characterize immune-mediated type 1 diabetes.[4] In a recent study in New South Wales, Australia, of 205 newly diagnosed patients with typical type 1 diabetes, 3.4% were negative for antipancreatic autoantibodies (ICA, IAA, GAD, IA-2) despite ongoing need for insulin.[5] In Japan, a rapid-onset insulin-deficient form of diabetes has been shown by pancreatic biopsies to be associated with a generalized lymphocytic infiltration of the pancreas and is presumed to be viral in origin.[6]

In the USA, many patients with non-immune type 1 diabetes may have what has been termed atypical diabetes mellitus (ADM) or 'flatbush' diabetes; this form of diabetes has been variously considered to be a form of type 1, type 2, or maturity-onset diabetes of the young.[1,7–9] This condition occurs throughout childhood with onset rarely past 40 years of age, and has only been described in African-American patients. It is not associated with HLA specificities. There is a strong family history in multiple generations giving a dominant pattern of inheritance. Although an individual patient may be overweight, reflecting the population prevalence of obesity, there is no association with obesity. There is an abnormal sex ratio with three times as many females as males being affected. Islet cell autoimmunity is absent. Although ketoacidosis is common at onset, insulin may not be required for survival after recovery from the acute metabolic deterioration; however, diabetic control may be poor and ketoacidosis may recur without insulin treatment in some individuals. There is no evidence of insulin resistance and insulin secretion is diminished but does not deteriorate.

Type 2 diabetes

Type 2 diabetes of childhood occurs predominantly during the second decade of life but is increasingly being described in prepubertal children. Obesity is almost always present with body mass index (BMI) above the 85–95th percentile for age and sex. Although seen in all races, there is much greater risk in African-American, Native American, Hispanic (especially Mexican) American, Asian, Pacific Islander, South Asian, Middle Eastern, and Australian Aborigine peoples.[10–22] There is no association with HLA specificities and a high percentage, probably greater than 75%, have first- or second-degree relatives affected. Sex ratios vary in different populations, from 4 to 6 females for every male in Native Americans to an even sex ratio in Libyan Arabs. Ketosis and ketoacidosis occur in one-third or more of newly diagnosed patients, resulting in frequent misclassification of type 2 diabetes as type 1 disease. Fatal complications of severe dehydration (hyperosmolar hyperglycemic coma, hypokalemia) may occur at the time of or before diagnosis.[23] Type 2 diabetes is often detected in the asymptomatic individual as a result of testing because of risk factors such as family history, or during routine school or sports examination. Other features of the insulin resistance syndrome are frequently present (Figure 2.2).

Autoantibody positive type 2 diabetes has long been recognized in adult populations with apparent type 2 diabetes and these individuals have been referred to as having either type 1.5 or, more commonly, latent autoimmune diabetes of adults (LADA). This is a phenomenon largely of younger adult patients, with 21% of 157 25–34 year olds in the United Kingdom Prospective Diabetes Study (UKPDS) being positive for ICA, 34% positive for GAD antibodies, and 20% positive for both, decreasing to 4%, 7%, and 2%, respectively, in the 1769 55–65 year olds.[24] The antibody-positive individuals were significantly less overweight than those who were antibody-negative and their HbA_{1c} concentrations were significantly higher. Furthermore, beta-cell function was significantly

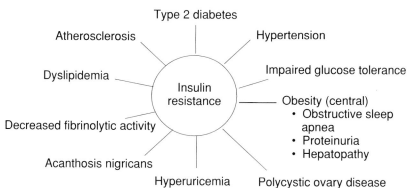

Figure 2.2 *The insulin resistance or metabolic syndrome.*[42]

decreased in antibody-positive individuals, particularly the younger patients, resulting in more rapid development of insulin dependence, typically 3 years following diagnosis. In a nationwide Swedish study of all 15–35-year-old newly diagnosed diabetes patients over a 2-year period ($n = 764$), 76% were classified as type 1, 14% as type 2, and the rest, unclassified. A remarkable 47% of type 2 patients and 59% of unclassified patients were positive for ICA, GAD antibodies, or IA-2.[25] In this study, as in the UKPDS, antibody positivity was associated with lighter body weight and lower C-peptide concentration.

As would be expected by the predominance of LADA among young adults thought to have type 2 diabetes, a substantial number of children with purported type 2 diabetes have been found to be antibody-positive. Among 48 children with type 2 diabetes, 8% demonstrated positivity for a fragment of islet cell antibody (ICA512), 30% were positive for GAD antibodies, and 35% for IAA.[26] Degree of obesity did not correlate with antibody positivity. As with type 1 diabetes, thyroid autoimmunity was present in several individuals with islet cell autoimmunity. In another study of 37 African-American children and adolescents with type 2 diabetes, 10.8% were positive for GAD antibodies, IA-2, or both.[27]

The presence of autoantibodies in patients clinically regarded as having type 2 diabetes is a dilemma in the classification of their diabetes. The question whether the presence of autoantibodies demands the classification of the patient as having type 1 diabetes is being debated. Diagnostic algorithms based on whether autoantibodies are present – therefore type 1 diabetes – or absent – therefore either maturity-onset diabetes of the young (MODY), idiopathic type 1 diabetes, or type 2 diabetes – have been proposed based on autoantibody and C-peptide levels. Although such algorithms may be helpful with most patients, there is increasing recognition of the group of patients who behave clinically as though they have type 2 diabetes but who have diabetes-specific autoantibodies. A unifying hypothesis (the accelerator hypothesis) has been proposed which suggests that the hyperglycemia secondary to insulin resistance is able to induce beta-cell apoptosis with the development of beta-cell autoimmunity.[28] Testing for ICA and GAD antibodies may be indicated in all pediatric patients thought to have type 2 diabetes, considering the high frequency of evidence of such autoimmunity in otherwise typical type 2 diabetes. The presence of such antibodies will indicate the need to check for thyroid autoimmunity and to consider other associated autoimmune disorders. Such testing will also provide therapeutic guidance, indicating the more likely deterioration of insulin secretion over the first few years from diagnosis.

Other specific types of diabetes

The eight subclassifications under this rubric include diabetes caused by:

1. genetic defects of beta-cell function
2. genetic defects in insulin action
3. diseases of the exocrine pancreas
4. endocrine disease, particularly glucocorticoid excess
5. drugs or chemicals
6. infections
7. uncommon forms of immune-mediated diabetes
8. other genetic syndromes associated with diabetes.

Genetic defects of beta-cell function (see Chapter 11)

Genetic defects of beta-cell function include mutations that result in MODY, mitochondrial mutations, and mutations that affect the insulin gene or affect cleavage of proinsulin.[29] The most important of these in the consideration of non-type-1 diabetes in children is MODY, defined as diabetes occurring before age 25, which is not insulin requiring, and not ketotic, with measurable C-peptide concentrations and absence of insulin requirement for 5 years after diagnosis, with an autosomal domi-nant pattern of transmission, although testing may be required to demonstrate this in milder forms. Affected families have been detected in Caucasian, Japanese, and South Asian populations.

The proportion of all diabetes that is due to MODY varies widely among different populations, from 0.14% in Germany to 3% in England and 4.8% in Madras, India, with one study indicating that 10% of Caucasian French families with type 2 diabetes have MODY. In a study of Japanese patients with type 1 diabetes, which is rare in this popula-tion, approx 6% had a molecular defect resulting in MODY. Molecular defects involving six genes have been identified in MODY families, with over 200 different mutations described.[30]

The rare mitochondrial mutations associated with diabetes and deaf-ness are, by definition, inherited from the mother who is always the source of the offspring's mitochondria. The most common mutation occurs at position 3243 of the mitochondrial gene encoding for leucine transfer RNA. Disease severity depends on the specific mutation, the pro-portion of normal and abnormal mitochondria, and their tissue distribu-tion.[31] Identical mitochondrial gene mutations may also be associated with syndromes, including myoclonic epilepsy, ragged red fiber disease, *m*itochondrial *e*ncephalopathy, *l*actic *a*cidosis, and *s*troke-like syndrome (MELAS syndrome).[32] The mitochondrial mutations interfere with beta-cell energy generation, impeding insulin secretion.

Genetic defects in insulin action

Numerous mutations in the insulin receptor have been described which are associated with dramatic insulin resistance, and are extremely rare.

Diseases of the exocrine pancreas

In the USA and Western Europe, cystic fibrosis (CF) is the most important pancreatic disorder associated with diabetes, which may resemble
type 1 or type 2 diabetes at various times in the same individual. With
increasing survival of CF patients, CF-related diabetes is becoming a substantial component of pediatric diabetes care. In Southeast Asia, thalassemia is a more common cause of secondary diabetes.

Endocrine disease

Cushing's syndrome, acromegaly, and pheochromocytoma have been
associated with secondary diabetes, as the result of pathologic counter-
regulation, with increased gluconeogenesis and peripheral insulin
resistance.

Drugs and chemicals

As with the endocrine disorders, treatment with glucocorticoids, growth
hormone, or catecholamines can be diabetogenic. A substantially
increased incidence of type 2 diabetes and impaired glucose tolerance
has been associated with growth hormone treatment of children and
adolescents.[33] Patients with acquired immunodeficiency receiving pen-
tamidine for pulmonary *Pneumocystis carinii* infection have developed
diabetes as the result of drug-induced beta-cell necrosis. Patients with
oncologic diseases may develop a reversible form of diabetes when on
various chemotherapy regimens, especially those combining high-dose
glucocorticoids and L-asparaginase.

Infection

The only infection for which there is incontrovertible proof that it
causes diabetes is congenital rubella. Approximately 10–15% of affected
individuals will develop diabetes in their lifetime.[34]

In severe infections of any kind, the stress and concomitant counter-
regulatory hormone production may result in stress hyperglycemia. In
very young patients, this may be prolonged and be accompanied by
ketosis or even ketoacidosis, particularly during a severe infection such
as meningitis. Because this state is not associated with specific damage to

the beta cells, the diabetes resolves with improvement in the infectious state.

Uncommon forms of immune-mediated diabetes

Anti-insulin receptor antibodies can result in severe insulin resistance. Affected individuals are lean and have acanthosis nigricans as a feature of their insulin resistance. Anti-insulin receptor autoantibodies typically produce hypoglycemia but glucose intolerance can also be seen.

Genetic syndromes associated with diabetes

Numerous syndromes are associated with diabetes, which in some instances appear related to obesity, such as with the Prader–Labhart–Willi syndrome and the Bardet–Biedl syndrome and, therefore, similar to isolated type 2 diabetes.[1]

Problems in classification

An analysis of about 700 newly diagnosed 5–19-year-old patients at the three university diabetes centers in Florida over the 5-year period from 1994–99 indicated that 3% of the approx 600 patients initially classified as type 1 diabetes were later considered to have type 2 disease and 8% of the approx 80 initially diagnosed as type 2 diabetes were later reclassified as type 1 disease.[35] This experience likely reflects the true proportion of patients in whom classification is challenging.

There are a number of reasons why the distinctions indicated in Table 2.3 may be problematic. With increasing obesity in childhood, as many as 20–25% of newly diagnosed patients who do not have type 2 diabetes may be overweight. Family history has low specificity because of the high frequency of type 2 diabetes in the population, with a random family history likelihood of approx 15%, and even greater in minority populations. Furthermore, a family history for type 2 diabetes is as much as three times more likely in patients with type 1 diabetes than in the general population and type 1 diabetes is more frequent in relatives of patients with type 2 diabetes.[36] The genetic interaction between type 1 and type 2 diabetes is also reflected in HLA haplotype interaction and, as

Table 2.3 Classification of the types of diabetes seen in children

Factor	Type 1	ADM	MODY	Type 2
Age at onset	throughout childhood	pubertal	pubertal	pubertal
Predominant race or ethnic distribution	all (low frequency in Asians)	African-American(AA)	Caucasian	Hispanic, AA, Native American
Onset	acute, severe	acute, severe	subtle	subtle to severe
Islet autoimmunity	present	absent	absent	absent
Insulin secretion	very low	moderately low	variable	decreased
Insulin sensitivity	normal (with BG control)	normal	normal	decreased
Ketosis, DKA at onset	up to 40%	common	rare	up to 33%
Obesity	as in population	as in population	uncommon	>90%
Proportion of diabetes	~80%[a]	>10%	<5%	~20%[a]
Percent of probands with affected 1° or 2° relative	5–10%	>75%	100%	~80%
Mode of inheritance	Non-Mendelian, generally sporadic	Autosomal dominant	Autosomal dominant	Non-Mendelian, strongly familial

[a] The proportion of pediatric diabetes patients having ADM, MODY, or type 2 diabetes will vary with racial/ethnic mix of the population; proportion of type 2 diabetes is increasing.

Source: Adapted from Winter et al.[29] and Rosenbloom et al.[31]

noted above, by the presence of diabetes-related autoimmunity markers in some children and adults with typical type 2 diabetes.[37] C-peptide measurements may be of limited help in differentiating type 1 and type 2 diabetes at onset and over the first year or so, because of the suppression of insulin secretion in type 2 diabetes at onset from glucotoxicity/lipotoxicity, and because normal C-peptide levels can be seen in the recovery phase of autoimmune diabetes (honeymoon phase).

Diagnostic strategy

Acute onset

Individuals with severe hyperglycemia or ketoacidosis, who are not obese, seldom require diagnostic reconsideration, unless they are African-American, with an autosomal dominant family history of diabetes in lean individuals before 40 years of age, in which case they likely have ADM. Obese patients with acute onset may require islet cell autoimmunity testing. Should this not be practical, or if there is acanthosis nigricans, the diagnosis can usually be made during the first several months on the basis of the ability to reduce insulin with weight reduction, exercise and, as necessary, response to oral hypoglycemic therapy.

Insidious onset or detection in the asymptomatic individual

Overweight individuals with mild but gradually progressive symptoms over months to years or who are asymptomatic can be considered to have type 2 diabetes. Lean individuals should have diabetes-related antibody studies which will indicate whether type 1 diabetes has been detected in an early stage. Absence of islet cell autoimmunity in a lean individual should lead to consideration of MODY. Fasting C-peptide concentrations may be of value after correction of hyperglycemia. Elevated levels indicate type 2 diabetes. Normal levels may reflect the recovery phase of type 1 diabetes, especially that detected early; repeat testing 1 year later will be more informative. The diagnosis may need to be reviewed in the context of the developing clinical picture and the results of further investigations.

Who to test for type 2 diabetes or prediabetes

Because testing is only a consideration for an at-risk population, rather than the population at large, in the context of secondary intervention, the activity can be considered to be case finding rather than screening, determination of obesity being the screening test. Case finding is justified when the condition tested for is sufficiently common to ratio-nalize the investment of resources, the condition is serious in terms of morbidity and mortality, there is a prolonged latency period without symptoms when abnormality can be detected, and a test is available that is sensitive (i.e., has few false negatives) and is accurate with acceptable specificity (i.e., with a minimal number of false positives). All of these criteria are readily met by type 2 diabetes in children and adolescents. The final criterion – that an intervention be available to prevent or delay disease onset or more effectively treat the condition detected when it is in the latency phase – is the most problematic.

A consensus panel of the ADA recommended that overweight chil-dren with two additional risk factors be considered for testing.[38] Overweight was defined as body mass index (BMI) >85th percentile for age and sex (Figures 2.3 and 2.4), weight for height >85th percentile, or weight >120% of ideal for height. The additional risk factors were a family history of type 2 diabetes in first- or second-degree relatives, race/ethnicity (Native American, African-American, Hispanic, Asian, Pacific Islander), and signs of insulin resistance or conditions associated with insulin resistance (acanthosis nigricans, hypertension, dyslipi-demia, ovarian hyperandrogenism). The age of initiation was suggested as 10 years or at the onset of puberty if puberty occurs at a younger age, with a frequency of retesting of every 2 years. The fasting plasma glucose was recommended as the preferred test.

There are a number of problems with these recommendations. They were developed without data and, in fact, many clinicians have detected asymptomatic diabetes in overweight patients who do not meet any of the additional criteria. The consensus panel provided an important dis-claimer that, 'Clinical judgment should be used to test for diabetes in

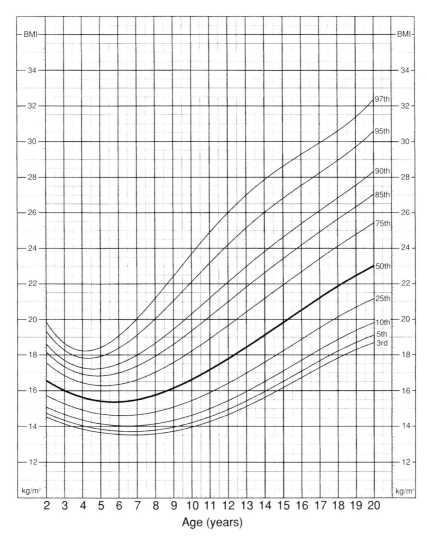

Figure 2.3 *Body mass index (BMI) percentiles for males (2–20 years) in the USA. Source: Developed by the National Center for Health Statistics in collaboration with the National Center for Chronic Disease Prevention and Health Promotion (2000).*

high-risk patients who do not meet these criteria'. Although type 2 diabetes is undoubtedly disproportionately seen in both adults and children from certain ethnic/racial groups, substantial numbers of white, non-Hispanic children, adolescents, and adults are also affected, making

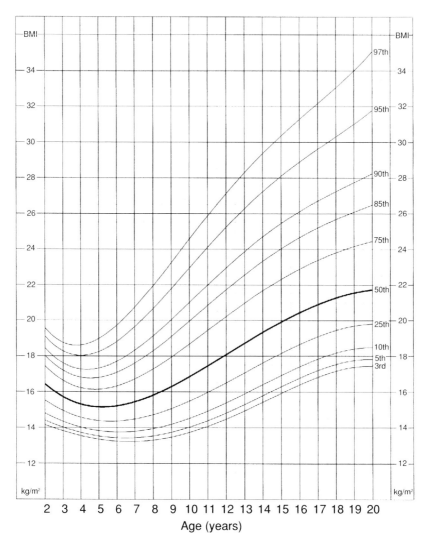

Figure 2.4 *Body mass index (BMI) percentiles for females (2–20 years) in the USA. Source: Developed by the National Center for Health Statistics in collaboration with the National Center for Chronic Disease Prevention and Health Promotion (2000).*

this a dubious criterion for testing. A recent report of testing a multiethnic cohort of 167 severely obese children and adolescents found IGT and silent type 2 diabetes in substantial numbers regardless of ethnicity.[39] Outside of North America, South Asian and Middle Eastern populations are also disproportionately at risk.[16,19,22] The age suggested is arbitrary, particularly with increasing numbers of obese youngsters under 10 years of age being seen with type 2 diabetes. The study noted above found that 25% of the 55 obese children aged 4–10 years had IGT, as did 21% of the 112 adolescents aged 11–18 years, whereas silent type 2 diabetes occurred in 4% of the adolescents.[39] The fasting plasma glucose was considered to be the most convenient test method by the consensus panel, but is unlikely to be sufficiently sensitive, because postprandial plasma glucose increases earlier during the course of development of type 2 diabetes.[40] A study in a large population of obese adults concluded that the fasting plasma glucose was a highly unreliable means of detecting type 2 diabetes compared to the 2-h post-glucose-load glucose level.[41]

Metabolic syndrome

Type 2 diabetes is now recognized as a manifestation of the metabolic syndrome, also known as the insulin resistance syndrome, the diabesity syndrome, or syndrome X, and this syndrome is increasingly being described in childhood and adolescence (see Figure 2.2).[42] A suggested definition includes glucose intolerance (IGT or diabetes) or insulin resistance (hyperinsulinemia), together with two or more of the following: hypertension, dyslipidemia, central adiposity, and microalbuminuria.[2] Several other components may be present but are not necessary for the diagnosis (hyperuricemia, coagulation disorders, raised PAI-1, polycystic ovary syndrome/ovarian hyperandrogenism). Acanthosis nigricans is frequently present.

Hypertension

Hypertension is an independent risk factor for the development of albuminuria, retinopathy, and cardiovascular disease in type 2 diabetes, estimated to account for 35–75% of diabetes complications.[43] Blood pressure is also an important factor in the early appearance of atherosclerotic lesions in children and adolescents.[44,45] Studies in adults have demonstrated a decrease in the incidence of major cardiovascular events with antihypertensive therapy.[46,47] In the UKPDS, hypertension control was more important in the reduction of cardiovascular events than was blood glucose control.[48]

Although no data are available for type 2 diabetes in children, a study of 589 children with type 1 diabetes onset before 17 years of age has demonstrated an increased risk of nephropathy, proliferative retinopathy, peripheral neuropathy, cardiovascular disease, and peripheral artery disease in the presence of elevated blood pressure during the first 10 years after diagnosis.[49] It is important to note that even modest elevations of blood pressure conferred increased risk; for example, systolic pressure 121–129 mmHg conferred a relative risk of cardiovascular disease of 2.5.

Blood pressure should be measured at each quarterly examination.[38] Blood pressure is obtained with the patient sitting; for children over the age of 13 years, the first and 5th Korotkov sounds (the point of disappearance of all sounds) should be recorded and measurement repeated at least twice to minimize the 'white coat effect'. (In children <13 years of age, the diastolic blood pressure can be recorded as the point of muffling of sounds (K4).) Elevations need to be rechecked at least twice at weekly intervals. Body size is the most important factor in blood pressure interpretation in children and adolescents. Tables 2.4 and 2.5 provide the 90th and 95th percentile references for blood pressure for each age in boys and girls in relationship to height percentiles.[50]

Dyslipidemia

Lipoprotein abnormalities in type 2 diabetes are extensive, and include hypertriglyceridemia, elevated very low-density lipoprotein (VLDL), elevated total and low-density lipoprotein (LDL) cholesterol, elevated lipoprotein(a), decreased high-density lipoprotein (HDL) cholesterol, increased small dense LDL particles, decreased lipoprotein lipase activity, increased lipoprotein glycation, and increased lipoprotein oxidation.[51] There are extensive studies demonstrating that the reduction of hyperlipidemia decreases the risk of coronary events in patients with diabetes, emphasizing the importance of monitoring and treating hyperlipidemia in children and adolescents with type 2 diabetes.

Table 2.4 Blood pressure levels for the 90th and 95th percentiles of blood pressure for females aged 1–17 years by percentiles of height

Age	Blood pressure percentile[b]	Systolic BP (mmHg) for height percentile[a]							Diastolic BP (mmHg) for height percentile[a]						
		5%	10%	25%	50%	75%	90%	95%	5%	10%	25%	50%	75%	90%	95%
1	90th	97	98	99	100	102	103	104	53	53	53	54	55	56	56
	95th	101	102	103	104	105	107	107	57	57	57	58	59	60	60
2	90th	99	99	100	102	103	104	105	57	57	58	58	59	60	61
	95th	102	103	104	105	107	108	109	61	61	62	62	63	64	65
3	90th	100	100	102	103	104	105	106	61	61	61	62	63	63	64
	95th	104	104	105	107	108	109	110	65	65	65	66	67	67	68
4	90th	101	102	103	104	106	107	108	63	63	64	65	65	66	67
	95th	105	106	107	108	109	111	111	67	67	68	69	69	70	71
5	90th	103	103	104	106	107	108	109	65	66	66	67	68	68	69
	95th	107	107	108	110	111	112	113	69	70	70	71	72	72	73
6	90th	104	105	106	107	109	110	111	67	67	68	69	69	70	71
	95th	108	109	110	111	112	114	114	71	71	72	73	73	74	75
7	90th	106	107	108	109	110	112	112	69	69	69	70	71	72	72
	95th	110	110	112	113	114	115	116	73	73	73	74	75	76	76

Table 2.4 Continued

Age	Blood pressure percentile[b]	Systolic BP (mmHg) for height percentile[a]							Diastolic BP (mmHg) for height percentile[a]						
		5%	10%	25%	50%	75%	90%	95%	5%	10%	25%	50%	75%	90%	95%
8	90th	108	109	110	111	112	113	114	70	70	71	71	72	73	74
	95th	112	112	113	115	116	117	118	74	74	75	75	76	77	78
9	90th	110	110	112	113	114	115	116	71	72	72	73	74	74	75
	95th	114	114	115	117	118	119	120	75	76	76	77	78	78	79
10	90th	112	112	114	115	116	117	118	73	73	73	74	75	76	76
	95th	116	116	117	119	120	121	122	77	77	77	78	79	80	80
11	90th	114	114	116	117	118	119	120	74	74	75	75	76	77	77
	95th	118	118	119	121	122	123	124	78	78	79	79	80	81	81
12	90th	116	116	118	119	120	121	122	75	75	76	76	77	78	78
	95th	120	120	121	123	124	125	126	79	79	80	80	81	82	82
13	90th	118	118	119	121	122	123	124	76	76	77	78	78	79	80
	95th	121	122	123	125	126	127	128	80	80	81	82	82	83	84
14	90th	119	120	121	122	124	125	126	77	77	78	79	79	80	81
	95th	123	124	125	126	128	129	130	81	81	82	83	83	84	85
15	90th	121	121	122	124	125	126	127	78	78	79	79	80	81	82
	95th	124	125	126	128	129	130	131	82	82	83	83	84	85	86

Table 2.4 Continued

Age	Blood pressure percentile[b]	Systolic BP (mmHg) for height percentile[a]							Diastolic BP (mmHg) for height percentile[a]						
		5%	10%	25%	50%	75%	90%	95%	5%	10%	25%	50%	75%	90%	95%
16	**90th**	122	122	123	125	126	127	128	79	79	79	80	81	82	82
	95th	125	126	127	128	130	131	132	83	83	83	84	85	86	86
17	**90th**	122	123	124	125	126	128	128	79	79	79	80	81	82	82
	95th	126	126	127	129	130	131	132	83	83	83	84	85	86	86

[a] Height percentile determined by standard growth curves.
[b] Blood pressure percentile determined by a single measurement.

Table 2.5 Blood pressure levels for the 90th and 95th percentiles of blood pressure for males aged 1–17 years by percentiles of height

Age	Blood pressure percentile[b]	Systolic BP (mmHg) for height percentile[a]							Diastolic BP (mmHg) for height percentile[a]						
		5%	10%	25%	50%	75%	90%	95%	5%	10%	25%	50%	75%	90%	95%
1	90th	94	95	97	98	100	102	102	50	51	52	53	54	54	55
	95th	98	99	101	102	104	106	106	55	55	56	57	58	59	59
2	90th	98	99	100	102	104	105	106	55	55	56	57	58	59	59
	95th	101	102	104	106	108	109	110	59	59	60	61	62	63	63
3	90th	100	101	103	105	107	108	109	59	59	60	61	62	63	63
	95th	104	105	107	109	111	112	113	63	63	64	65	66	67	67
4	90th	102	103	105	107	109	110	111	62	62	63	64	65	66	66
	95th	106	107	109	111	113	114	115	66	67	67	68	69	70	71
5	90th	104	105	106	108	110	112	112	65	65	66	67	68	69	69
	95th	108	109	110	112	114	115	116	69	70	70	71	72	73	74
6	90th	105	106	108	110	111	113	114	67	68	69	70	70	71	72
	95th	109	110	112	114	115	117	117	72	72	73	74	75	76	76
7	90th	106	107	109	111	113	114	115	69	70	71	72	72	73	74
	95th	110	111	113	115	116	118	119	74	74	75	76	77	78	78

Table 2.5 Continued

Age	Blood pressure percentile[b]	Systolic BP (mmHg) for height percentile[a]							Diastolic BP (mmHg) for height percentile[a]						
		5%	10%	25%	50%	75%	90%	95%	5%	10%	25%	50%	75%	90%	95%
8	90th	107	108	110	112	114	115	116	71	71	72	73	74	75	75
	95th	111	112	114	116	118	119	120	75	76	76	77	78	79	80
9	90th	109	110	112	113	115	117	117	72	73	73	74	75	76	77
	95th	113	114	116	117	119	121	121	76	77	78	79	80	80	81
10	90th	110	112	113	115	117	118	119	73	74	74	75	76	77	78
	95th	114	115	117	119	121	122	123	77	78	79	80	80	81	82
11	90th	112	113	115	117	119	120	121	74	74	75	76	77	78	78
	95th	116	117	119	121	123	124	125	78	79	79	80	81	82	83
12	90th	115	116	117	119	121	123	123	75	75	76	77	78	78	79
	95th	119	120	121	123	125	126	127	79	79	80	81	82	83	83
13	90th	117	118	120	122	124	125	126	75	76	76	77	78	79	80
	95th	121	122	124	126	128	129	130	79	80	81	82	83	83	84
14	90th	120	121	123	125	126	128	128	76	76	77	78	79	80	80
	95th	124	125	127	128	130	132	132	80	81	81	82	83	84	85
15	90th	123	124	125	127	129	131	131	77	77	78	79	80	81	81
	95th	127	128	129	131	133	134	135	81	82	83	83	84	85	86

Table 2.5 *Continued*

Age	Blood pressure percentile[b]	Systolic BP (mmHg) for height percentile[a]							Diastolic BP (mmHg) for height percentile[a]						
		5%	10%	25%	50%	75%	90%	95%	5%	10%	25%	50%	75%	90%	95%
16	90th	125	126	128	130	132	133	134	79	79	80	81	82	82	83
	95th	129	130	132	134	136	137	138	83	83	84	85	86	87	87
17	90th	128	129	131	133	134	136	136	81	81	82	83	84	85	85
	95th	132	133	135	136	138	140	140	85	85	86	87	88	89	89

[a] Height percentile determined by standard growth curves.
[b] Blood pressure percentile determined by a single measurement.

Acanthosis nigricans

Acanthosis nigricans (AN) is considered a hallmark of insulin resistance, typically seen in obesity, but also in lean individuals with genetic insulin resistance syndromes. There is wide ethnic variability in frequency of AN with obesity: approx 90% of obese Native Americans, approx 50% of obese African-Americans, approx 15% of obese Hispanic Americans, and fewer than 5% of obese white youngsters have AN.[52] AN also has varying specificity as an indicator of hyperinsulinism, inversely to its frequency of association with obesity. It is associated with IGT or type 2 diabetes in approx 25% of those under 20 years of age and approx 45% of those 20–30 years old.[52] In a study of 139 overweight African-American and white 6–10 year olds, AN was not considered to be a reliable marker for hyperinsulinism.[53]

References

1. The Expert Committee on the Diagnosis and Classification of Diabetes Mellitus. Report of the Expert Committee on the Diagnosis and Classification of Diabetes Mellitus. *Diabetes Care* 2001; **24**:S5–20.
2. World Health Organization. Definition, diagnosis and classification of diabetes mellitus and its complications. Report of a WHO Consultation. Part 1: Diagnosis and classification of diabetes mellitus. 1999 WHO/NCD/NCS/99.2.
3. Tuomilehto J, Lindstrom J, Valle TT *et al.* for the Finnish Diabetes Prevention Study Group. Prevention of type 2 diabetes mellitus by changes in lifestyle among subjects with impaired glucose tolerance. *N Engl J Med* 2001; **344**:1345–50.
4. Ko GT, Chan JC, Yeung VT *et al.* Antibodies to glutamic acid decarboxylase in young Chinese diabetic patients. *Ann Clin Biochem* 1998; **35**:761–7.
5. Craig ME. Studies in the epidemiology and pathogenesis of type 1 diabetes. PhD thesis, University of Sydney, 2001, p 176.
6. Imagawa A, Hanafusa T, Miyagawa J, Matsuzawa Y. A novel subtype of type 1 diabetes mellitus characterized by a rapid onset and an absence of diabetes-related antibodies. Osaka IDDM Study Group. *N Engl J Med* 2000; **342**:301–7.
7. Winter WE, Maclaren NK, Riley WJ *et al.* Maturity onset diabetes of youth in black Americans. *N Engl J Med* 1987; **316**:285–91.
8. Banerji MA, Chaiken RL, Huey H *et al.* GAD antibody negative NIDDM in adult black subjects with diabetic ketoacidosis and increased frequency of human leukocyte antigen DR3 and DR4. Flatbush diabetes. *Diabetes* 1994; **43**:741–5.
9. Banerji MA. Impaired beta-cell and alpha-cell function in African-American children with type 2 diabetes mellitus – 'Flatbush diabetes'. *J Pediatr Endocrinol Metab* 2002; **15**(suppl 1):493–501.

10. Dabelea D, Hanson RL, Bennett PH *et al*. Increasing prevalence of type 2 diabetes in American Indian children. *Diabetologia* 1998; **41**:904–10.
11. Dean HJ. NIDDM-Y in First Nation children in Canada. *Clin Pediatr* 1998; **39**:89–96.
12. Glaser NS, Jones KL. Non-insulin-dependent diabetes mellitus in Mexican-American children. *West J Med* 1998; **168**:11–16.
13. Pinhas-Hamiel O, Dolan LM, Daniels SR *et al*. Increased incidence of non-insulin-dependent diabetes mellitus among adolescents. *J Pediatr* 1996; **128**:608–15.
14. Scott CR, Smith JM, Cradock MM, Pihoker C. Characteristics of youth-onset non-insulin-dependent diabetes mellitus at diagnosis. *Pediatrics* 1997; **100**:84–91.
15. Neufeld ND, Raffal LF, Landon C *et al*. Early presentation of type 2 diabetes in Mexican-American youth. *Diabetes Care* 1998; **21**:80–6.
16. Kadiki OA, Reddy MR, Marzouk AA. Incidence of insulin-dependent diabetes (IDDM) and non-insulin-dependent diabetes (NIDDM) (0–34 years at onset) in Benghazi, Libya. *Diabetes Res Clin Pract* 1996; **32**:165–73.
17. Chan JCN, Cheung CK, Swaminathan R *et al*. Obesity, albuminuria, and hypertension among Hong Kong Chinese with non-insulin-dependent diabetes mellitus (NIDDM). *Postgrad Med J* 1993; **69**:204–10.
18. Kitagawa T, Owada M, Urakami T, Yamauchi K. Increased incidence of non-insulin dependent diabetes mellitus among Japanese schoolchildren correlates with an increased intake of animal protein and fat. *Clin Pediatr* 1998; **37**:111–15.
19. Sayeed MA, Hussain MZ, Banu A *et al*. Prevalence of diabetes in a suburban population of Bangladesh. *Diabetes Res Clin Pract* 1997; **34**:149–55.
20. Braun B, Zimmerman MB, Kretchmer N *et al*. Risk factors for diabetes and cardiovascular disease in young Australian aborigines. A 5-year follow-up study. *Diabetes Care* 1996; **19**:472–9.
21. McGrath NM, Parker GN, Dawson P. Early presentation of type 2 diabetes mellitus in young New Zealand Maori. *Diabetes Res Clin Pract* 1999; **43**:205–9.
22. Ehtisham S, Barrett TG, Shawl NJ. Type 2 diabetes mellitus in UK children – an emerging problem. *Diabetic Med* 2000; **17**:867–71.
23. Morales A, Rosenbloom AL. Death at the onset of type 2 diabetes (T2DM) in African-American youth. *Pediatr Res* 2002; **51**:124A.
24. Turner R, Stratton I, Horton V *et al*. for UK Prospective Diabetes Study (UKPDS) Group. UKPDS 25: autoantibodies to islet cell cytoplasm and glutamic acid decarboxylase for prediction of insulin requirement in type 2 diabetes. *Lancet* 1997; **350**:1288–93.
25. Landin-Olsson M. Latent autoimmune diabetes in adults. *Ann NY Acad Sci* 2002; **958**:112–16.
26. Hathout EH, Thomas W, El-Shahawy M *et al*. Diabetic autoimmune markers in children and adolescents with type 2 diabetes. *Pediatrics* 2001; **107**:e102.
27. Umpaichitra V, Banerji MA, Castells S. Autoantibodies in children with type 2 diabetes mellitus. *J Pediatr Endocrinol Metab* 2002; **15**:525–30.
28. Wilkin TJ. The accelerator hypothesis. *Diabetologia* 2001; **44**:914–22.
29. Winter WE, Nakamura M, House DV. Monogenic diabetes mellitus in youth: the MODY syndromes. *Endocrinol Metab Clin N Am* 1999; **28**:765–85.

30. Doria A, Plengvidhya N. Recent advances in the genetics of maturity onset diabetes of the young and other forms of autosomal dominant diabetes. *Curr Opin Endocrinol Diabetes* 2000; **7**:203–10.
31. Rosenbloom AL, Joe JR, Young RS, Winter WE. The emerging epidemic of type 2 diabetes mellitus in youth. *Diabetes Care* 1999; **22**:345–54.
32. Strachan J, McLellan A, Kirkpatrick M *et al*. Ketoacidosis: an unusual presentation of MELAS. *J Inherited Metab Dis* 2001; **24**:409–10.
33. Cutfield WS, Wilton P, Bennmarker H *et al*. Incidence of diabetes mellitus and impaired glucose tolerance in children and adolescents receiving growth hormone treatment. *Lancet* 2000; **355**:610–13.
34. McIntosh ED, Menser MA. A fifty-year follow-up of congenital rubella. *Lancet* 1992; **340** (8816):414–15.
35. Macaluso CJ, Bauer UE, Deeb LC *et al*. Type 2 diabetes mellitus among Florida children and adolescents, 1994 through 1998. *Public Health Rep* 2002; **117**:373–9.
36. Dahlquist G, Blom L, Tuvemo T *et al*. The Swedish childhood diabetes study – results from a nine-year case register and a one-year case-referent study indicating that type 1 (insulin-dependent) diabetes mellitus is associated with both type 2 (non-insulin-dependent) diabetes mellitus and autoimmune disorders. *Diabetologia* 1989; **32**:2–6.
37. Li H, Lindholm E, Almgren P *et al*. Possible human leukocyte antigen-mediated genetic interaction between type 1 and type 2 diabetes. *J Clin Endocrinol Metab* 2001; **86**:574–82.
38. American Diabetes Association. Type 2 diabetes in children and adolescents: consensus conference report. *Diabetes Care* 2000; **23**:381–9.
39. Sinha R, Fisch G, Teague B *et al*. Prevalence of impaired glucose tolerance among children and adolescents with marked obesity. *N Engl J Med* 2002; **346**:802–10.
40. DeFronzo RA. Lilly Lecture. The triumvirate: beta cell, muscle, liver. A collusion responsible for NIDDM. *Diabetes* 1988; **37**:667–87.
41. Richard JL, Sultan A, Daures J-P *et al*. Diagnosis of diabetes mellitus and intermediate glucose abnormalities in obese patients based on ADA (1997) and WHO (1985) criteria. *Diabetic Med* 2002; **19**:292–9.
42. American Diabetes Association Consensus Development Conference On Insulin Resistance. *Diabetes Care* 1998; **21**:310–14.
43. Gall M-A, Rossing P, Skott P *et al*. Prevalence of micro and macroalbuminuria, arterial hypertension, retinopathy and large vessel disease in European type 2 (non-insulin dependent) diabetes mellitus. *Diabetologia* 1991; **34**:655–61.
44. Berenson GS, Srinivasan SR, Bao W *et al*. Association between multiple cardiovascular risk factors and atherosclerosis in children and young adults. The Bogalusa Heart Study. *N Engl J Med* 1998; **338**:1650–6.
45. Malcom GT, Oalmann MC, Strong JP. Risk factors for atherosclerosis in young subjects: the PDAY Study. Pathobiological Determinants of Atherosclerosis in Youth. *Ann NY Acad Sci* 1997; **817**:179–88.
46. Heart Outcome Prevention Evaluation (HOPE) Study Investigators. Effects of ramipril on cardiovascular and microvascular outcomes in people with diabetes mellitus. *Lancet* 2000; **255**:253–9.
47. Hansson L, Zanchetti A, Carruthers SG *et al*. for the HOT Study Group. Effects of intensive blood-pressure lowering and low-dose aspirin in patients with

hypertension: principal results of the Hypertension Optimal Treatment (HOT) randomized trial. *Lancet* 1998; **351**:1755–62.

48. UKPDS Group. Tight blood pressure control and risk of macrovascular and microvascular complications in type 2 diabetes: UKPDS 38. *Br Med J* 1998; **317**:703–13.

49. Orchard TJ, Forrest KYZ, Kuller LH, Becker DJ. Lipid and blood pressure treatment goals for type 1 diabetes: 10 year incidence data from the Pittsburgh Epidemiology of Complications Study. *Diabetes Care* 2001; **24**:1053–9.

50. Rosner B, Prineas RJ, Loggie JM, Daniels SR. Blood pressure nomograms for children and adolescents, by height, sex, and age, in the United States. *J Pediatr* 1993; **123**:871–86.

51. Goldberg IJ. Diabetic dyslipidemia: causes and consequences. *J Clin Endocrinol Metab* 2001; **86**:965–71.

52. Stuart CA, Gilkison CR, Smith MM *et al.* Acanthosis nigricans as a risk factor for non-insulin dependent diabetes mellitus. *Clin Pediatr* 1998; **37**:73–80.

53. Nguyen TT, Keil MF, Russell DL *et al.* Relation of acanthosis nigricans to hyperinsulinemia and insulin sensitivity in overweight African-American and white children. *J Pediatr* 2001; **138**:474–80.

chapter 3

Type 2 diabetes in children and adolescents in North America

Giuseppina Imperatore, Desmond E Williams, and Frank Vinicor

Introduction

Traditionally, diabetes mellitus in youth was thought to be almost esclusively type 1 diabetes, but there have been increasing numbers of reports of type 2 diabetes among youth in the last 30 years. In 1971, Dr Harvey Knowles wrote:

> A second type of diabetes in young persons closely resembles that of the stable middle-aged onset type. Herein the patients as a rule have no symptoms, are overweight, can secrete insulin, and respond to sulfonylurea therapy. Often the diagnosis is made serendipitously. In the Juvenile Diabetic Clinic at the Cincinnati General Hospital 11 of these patients have been followed along with 300 patients with the unstable insulin deficient type of diabetes. The age of these 11 patients at diagnosis ranged from 11 to 17 years. The prevalence of this type of diabetes very likely is higher than presently appreciated, because of lack of symptoms or signs leading to suspicion of diabetes.[1]

Type 2 diabetes is increasingly being reported, especially in minority populations.[2-6] Type 2 diabetes has been reported in youth from the United Kingdom,[5,6] Japan,[7,8] Hong Kong,[9] Bangladesh,[10] Libya,[11] Australia,[12] and New Zealand.[13]

Despite these recent reports, our understanding of the magnitude of various types of diabetes in young people from different populations remains limited. Furthermore, there is no 'gold standard' for differentiating the types of childhood diabetes. Many of the existing methods have relied on such clinical factors as age at onset, obesity, family history, acuteness of onset, and insulin therapy, but these factors do not reliably differentiate the types. For example, adolescents with type 2 diabetes can present with diabetic ketoacidosis (DKA), and patients with type 1 diabetes may be obese and not have severe acute symptoms at the time of diagnosis. Misclassification may result in improper disease management, which is one reason for the need to develop reliable and valid classifications of diabetes. Such taxonomy should:

1. differentiate the types of diabetes in children and adolescents
2. be suitable for estimating the frequency of the types of diabetes in various populations
3. provide effective classification(s) for clinical diagnosis, research studies, and population surveillance.

In this chapter, we review what is known about the epidemiology of diabetes in youth, including the magnitude of the problem and its risk factors and we highlight gaps in our knowledge and the challenges for public health.

Prevalence and incidence

A high frequency of type 2 diabetes in adolescents was initially reported in Pima Indians.[2] Diabetes is highly prevalent in the Pima Indian population, and is almost always type 2 diabetes, even when it occurs at a young age.[14,15] A recent analysis that included data on 5274 Pima Indian children aged less than 20 years reported a strong increase in the prevalence of type 2 diabetes from 1967–76 to 1987–96.[16] Among 15–19 year olds, the prevalence of type 2 diabetes increased in boys from 2.4% to 3.8% and in girls from 2.7% to 5.3%. Since 1981, the Indian Health Service (IHS) has collected data on reported diabetes from outpatient clinics serving American Indian populations. Prevalence estimates from these data for youths aged 15–19 years were 3.2 per 1000 in 1990 and 5.4 per 1000 in 1998.[17] The magnitude of the problem in other major ethnic or racial groups is not known. A report from a major pediatric center in Cincinnati (Ohio) was the first to estimate the incidence rates for type 2 diabetes in 10- to 19-year-old African-American and white children, based on projections from the referral population. The incidence of diagnosed type 2 diabetes increased from 0.7 per 100,000 in 1982 to 7.2 per 100,000 in 1994.[18] There is also indirect evidence from US population-based registries of type 1 diabetes that the incidence of type 2 diabetes may be increasing among youth. According to reports from the US registry of type 1 diabetes in Allegheny County, Pennsylvania, the annual incidence of diagnosed diabetes mellitus (based on insulin treatment started at diagnosis) among 15- to 19-year-old African-Americans increased from 13.8 per 100,000 in 1985–89 to 30.4 per 100,000 in 1990–94.[19] This increase may have been partially attributable to an increase in type 2 diabetes, which could have been misclassified as type 1 diabetes and treated with insulin at diagnosis. Data from the Chicago, Illinois type 1 diabetes registry also support this hypothesis. Indeed, after reviewing medical records and interviewing patients listed in the Chicago registry, Lipton *et al.*[20] identified a subset with clinical characteristics resembling type 2 diabetes. They found that among African-American and Hispanic children aged 0–17 years the annual incidence of presumed type 2 diabetes increased by 9% from 1985 to 1994, a period in which the incidence of type 1 diabetes remained unchanged.[20]

Until 1992, type 2 diabetes accounted for 2–4% of all newly diagnosed cases of diabetes under the age of 19 years. In the last decade, however, this proportion ranged from 8% to 45%, with considerable variation by age and race/ethnicity.[21]

Part of the secular increase of type 2 diabetes may be attributed to greater awareness that led to more diagnosis, but clinical recommendations for screening youth for type 2 diabetes were not published until 2000.[22] Moreover, better diagnosis cannot explain the trends observed in population-based studies, and as noted above, the presence of a small proportion of patients with type 2 diabetes has long been recognized in pediatric populations.[1] Even with the great increase reported, the presence of type 2 diabetes in youth might be very much underestimated. In the USA, there is one undiagnosed adult with type 2 diabetes for every two or three diagnosed adults,[23] and this might also well be the case among children and adolescents.

Clinical characteristics

A review of 578 cases of type 2 diabetes in youth found that about 94% were from minority communities.[24] The mean age at diagnosis usually coincided with the age of puberty (approximately 12–14 years), except among the Pima Indians, where the mean age at diagnosis was 16 years. Type 2 diabetes was rarely observed in children under 10 years of age, although in the Pima population it occurred as early as 4 years of age. The disease was more common in girls than in boys, with ratios ranging from 2:1 to 6:1. It was found that 74–95% of the cases had a first- or second-degree relative with diabetes.

Obesity and acanthosis nigricans, both strongly related to insulin resistance, were common. In Cincinnati, 66% of the children with type 2 diabetes were referred because of symptoms or acute illness, and 32% because of glycosuria during routine testing.[18] Weight loss and ketosis were common, and ketoacidosis was also reported. In type 2 diabetes among those less then 20 years, data on complications are scarce.

Among 114 adolescents with type 2 diabetes who had a mean age at diagnosis of 15.5 years, and were identified by the diabetes registry of a health management organization, 26% had hypertension (defined as systolic or diastolic blood pressure >90th age-, gender-, and height-specific percentile, or the use of antihypertensives) and glycated hemoglobin concentration (HbA_{1c}) averaged 9%.[25]

The incidence of microvascular complications was assessed in Pima Indians who were diagnosed with type 2 diabetes before the age of 20 years.[26] By the age of 30 years 57% had developed nephropathy (defined as protein-to-creatinine ratio ≥ 0.5 g protein per g creatinine) and 45% developed retinopathy (defined as the presence of at least one microaneurysm, hemorrhage, or proliferative retinopathy).

In Manitoba and northwestern Ontario, among young adults whose type 2 diabetes was diagnosed before the age of 17 years, 63% had an HbA$_{1c}$ concentration above 10% and 6.3% were on dialysis.[27] All these findings indicate that a high prevalence and lifetime incidence of microvascular and macrovascular complications are likely among young adults who develop type 2 diabetes during childhood. Delayed diagnosis, poor glucose control, and the presence of risk factors for cardiovascular disease during the teenage years, and the long duration of diabetes may all predispose to early complications. In adults, diabetes control is insufficient to prevent or delay complications,[28] and this situation may be worse for children and adolescents. Adolescents may be particularly reluctant to undertake self-management and keep follow-up appointments, and they may experience behavioral problems; access to health care may also be inadequate. Thus, carefully conducted studies of the quality of care and of potential interventions among children are needed.

Major risk factors and their secular trends

Type 2 diabetes results from the interaction between genetic and environmental factors. The genetic contribution, as highlighted in Chapter 11, likely involves several gene variants, each with relatively modest effect, that interact with each other or with environmental factors resulting in disease. The discussion below focuses on modifiable factors that have been linked to an increased risk of developing type 2 diabetes.

Prenatal, perinatal, and early life factors

Associations between both low and high birth weight and type 2 diabetes in children have been described in many populations.[29] The increased risk associated with high birth weight is largely explained by maternal diabetes during pregnancy.[29] Results from animal models indicate that the exposure to diabetes *in utero* results in defects in both insulin action and insulin secretion, leading to the development of diabetes later in life.[30] Data from the Pima Indian study demonstrate that within the same family, children born after a mother's diagnosis of diabetes have a much greater risk of developing diabetes at an early age than children born before the diagnosis.[31] Because the offspring born before and after the onset of their mother's diabetes carry a similar risk of inheriting the mother's diabetes susceptibility genes, the difference in risk reflects the effect of intrauterine exposure to hyperglycemia. This observation has important public health implications, indicating a cumulative effect of women developing diabetes during childbearing age and exposing their children to diabetes *in utero*, thereby increasing the risk to the offspring of developing diabetes at a younger age.

Low birth weight has also been associated with type 2 diabetes and insulin resistance in childhood.[15,32–34] Fetal programming in response to the in-utero environment,[35,36] the influence of genetic factors on both intrauterine growth and glucose tolerance later in life,[37,38] and the selective survival of small babies genetically predisposed to type 2 diabetes and insulin resistance[29] may all be responsible for this association.

Breast-feeding reduces the risk of both type 2 diabetes and obesity in children,[39–41] with a dose–response relationship between the duration of breast-feeding and protection from type 2 diabetes and obesity.[39,41,42] This is encouraging, because the US Pregnancy Risk Assessment Monitoring System 1993–99 showed a significant positive trend in breast-feeding at 4 weeks in all but four states studied.[43]

Obesity

In the United States the rate of overweight among children has dramatically increased over the past 25 years,[44] and obesity is a well-established risk factor for the development of type 2 diabetes in adults. Results from the US 1999–2000 National Health and Nutrition Examination Survey (NHANES) indicate that approx. 15% of children aged 6–11 years and of adolescents aged 12–19 years are obese (defined as a body mass index greater than or equal to the age- and sex-specific 95th percentile)[44] (Figure 3.1). This represents an increase of 5 percentage points between NHANES III conducted in 1988–94 and NHANES 1999–2000. It is also apparent that obesity prevalence in children and adolescents was relatively stable from the 1960s to the early 1980s (Figure 3.1); from NHANES II (1976–80) to NHANES III, however, obesity prevalence nearly doubled

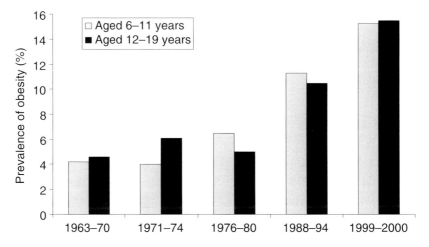

Figure 3.1 *Gender- and age-specific BMI (body mass index) > the 95th percentile. Source: National Health Examination Survey (NHES), National Health and Nutrition Examination Survey (NHANES).*

among both children and adolescents. Coinciding with this trend, frequency of type 2 diabetes increased among youth. The Pima Indian prospective study showed that the mean weight of Pima Indian children increased significantly between the periods of 1967–76 and 1987–96, and the prevalence of type 2 diabetes increased significantly with increasing relative weight.[16] Dietary changes and reduction in physical activity are considered the underlying cause of this obesity epidemic in youth.

Diet

During the last 30 years, the diets of American children and adolescents have undergone considerable changes. The NHANES surveys show that among US adolescents the proportion of total calories represented by fats declined from 37% to 33% between the early 1970s and the early 1990s.[45] During the same period, the proportion of calories from saturated fatty acids declined from 14% to 12%. Although these data indicate that fat intake of US children changed favorably over two decades or so, they also indicate that children in the early 1990s were still consuming more than the contemporary dietary recommendations for total fat ($\leq$ 30% of energy) and saturated fatty acids ($\leq$ 10% of energy). Because dietary fat intake has decreased, the apparent slight increase in mean energy intake (95 kcal/day from NHANES I to NHANES III, albeit a change in methodology makes comparisons difficult[45]) among adolescents aged 12–19 years most likely came from carbohydrate intake, especially from refined foods such as breads, pizza, cakes, cookies, high fat potatoes, and soft drinks.[45,46] Soft drinks supply as much as 8% of total energy intake of US adolescents,[45] and among children 11–18, soft drink consumption more than doubled from 1965 to 1996.[46] These high glycemic-index foods produce greater increases in blood glucose concentrations in the postprandial phase than do foods with a low glycemic index,[47] and a high glycemic-index diet has been associated with type 2 diabetes in adults.[48–50]

Physical activity

Physical activity may play an important role in the trends observed in obesity and may also have an effect on insulin resistance that is independent of its relationship with obesity.[51–55] The US 2001 Youth Risk Behavior Surveillance (YRBS), conducted among a nationally representative sample of high school students, found that about a quarter of boys and more than a third of girls had not participated in vigorous or moderate physical activities during the preceding week.[56] The proportion of inactive adolescents increased with age and, of particular concern, girls were more likely to be physically inactive than were boys in all age groups.[56] A recent prospective study of girls followed from age of 9 or 10 to 18 or 19 years confirm this trend.[57] Moreover, consistent with the increase in obesity among adolescents, only about a half of US high school students regularly attend physical education classes, and this proportion has not increased during the past 10 years.[56] The 2001 YRBS showed that about 40% of boys and 35% of girls watch 3 or more hours of TV per day.[56]

Conclusions

In the 1990s, type 2 diabetes in children was recognized as an emerging public health problem in North America.[22,24] The American Diabetes

Association and the American Academy of Pediatrics issued a joint consensus statement to help health care providers in diagnosing, classifying, and treating type 2 diabetes in children.[22] Still, several important pieces of the puzzle with significant clinical and public health implications are missing. First, we need to develop better case definition(s) that will differentiate between types of diabetes in children and will be suitable for population studies and for clinical diagnosis. Secondly, epidemiological data on the magnitude of the problem, its secular trends, and natural history are needed for several at-risk populations. In the United States these issues are currently being investigated in the SEARCH for Diabetes in Youth study sponsored by the Centers for Disease Control and Prevention and the National Institutes of Health. Well-coordinated multicenter trials testing the feasibility of reducing multiple risk factors in children and their benefits on health outcomes are also needed.

Among adults, type 2 diabetes is highly related to behavioral and environmental factors. Three major randomized controlled trials conducted in diverse countries, settings, and populations, confirm that effective lifestyle intervention can prevent or delay progression to type 2 diabetes among overweight adults with impaired glucose tolerance (a 2 h 75 g post-load glucose 7.8–11.1 mmol/l).[50,58,59] Although the efficacy of these interventions in children is unknown, it would be surprising if they were not at least as successful in young persons. These interventions would have to be family-based and include policy changes in schools that address diet and physical activity.[60] Community-based efforts are important for controlling childhood obesity and preventing diabetes and to encourage lifelong patterns of positive health behaviors.

Despite the availability of effective treatment, the quality of care for adult type 2 diabetes remains suboptimal,[28] and this situation is likely to be worse for children and adolescents.[21,24] Thus, carefully conducted studies of quality of care and of potential management options among children are needed. Finally, type 2 diabetes in children offers some exceptional opportunities to understand the causes of the disease and of insulin resistance, with the benefit of developing better primary prevention.

The emergence of type 2 diabetes in young people epitomizes the growing problem of chronic diseases worldwide and their extension to youth. The rising prevalence of obesity and type 2 diabetes in children is also the consequence of worldwide social and economic changes. To fight type 2 diabetes as a pediatric disease will require use of recent medical advances, but will also require understanding and questioning of the untoward health changes brought from industrialization.

References

1. Knowles HC Jr. Diabetes mellitus in childhood and adolescence. *Med Clin North Am* 1971; **55**:975–87.
2. Savage PJ, Bennett PH, Senter RG *et al*. High prevalence of diabetes in young Pima Indians: evidence of phenotypic variation in a genetically isolated population. *Diabetes* 1979; **28**:937–42.
3. Young TK, McIntyre LL, Dooley J *et al*. Epidemiologic features of diabetes mellitus among Indians in northwestern Ontario and northeastern Manitoba. *Can Med Assoc J* 1985; **132**:793–7.
4. Dean H, Moffatt ME. Prevalence of diabetes mellitus among Indian children in Manitoba. *Arctic Med Res* 1988; **47**(Suppl 1):532–4.
5. Ehtisham S, Barrett TG, Shaw NJ. Type 2 diabetes mellitus in UK children – an emerging problem. *Diabet Med* 2000; **17**:867–71.
6. Drake AJ, Smith A, Betts PR *et al*. Type 2 diabetes in obese white children. *Arch Dis Child* 2002; **86**:207–8.
7. Kitagawa T, Owada M, Urakami T *et al*. Increased incidence of non-insulin dependent diabetes mellitus among Japanese schoolchildren correlates with an increased intake of animal protein and fat. *Clin Pediatr (Phila)* 1998; **37**:111–15.
8. Owada M, Hanaoka Y, Tanimoto Y *et al*. Descriptive epidemiology of non-insulin dependent diabetes mellitus detected by urine glucose screening in school children in Japan. *Acta Paediatr Jpn* 1990; **32**:716–24.
9. Chan JC, Cheung CK, Swaminathan R *et al*. Obesity, albuminuria and hypertension among Hong Kong Chinese with non-insulin-dependent diabetes mellitus (NIDDM). *Postgrad Med J* 1993; **69**:204–10.
10. Sayeed MA, Hussain MZ, Banu A *et al*. Prevalence of diabetes in a suburban population of Bangladesh. *Diabetes Res Clin Pract* 1997; **34**:149–55.
11. Kadiki OA, Reddy MR, Marzouk AA. Incidence of insulin-dependent diabetes (IDDM) and non-insulin-dependent diabetes (NIDDM) (0–34 years at onset) in Benghazi, Libya. *Diabetes Res Clin Pract* 1996; **32**:165–73.
12. Braun B, Zimmermann MB, Kretchmer N *et al*. Risk factors for diabetes and cardiovascular disease in young Australian aborigines. A 5-year follow-up study. *Diabetes Care* 1996; **19**:472–9.
13. McGrath NM, Parker GN, Dawson P. Early presentation of type 2 diabetes mellitus in young New Zealand Maori. *Diabetes Res Clin Pract* 1999; **43**:205–9.

14. Knowler WC, Bennett PH, Bottazzo GF *et al*. Islet cell antibodies and diabetes mellitus in Pima Indians. *Diabetologia* 1979; **17**:161–4.
15. Dabelea D, Palmer JP, Bennett PH *et al*. Absence of glutamic acid decarboxylase antibodies in Pima Indian children with diabetes mellitus. *Diabetologia* 1999; **42**:1265–6.
16. Dabelea D, Hanson RL, Bennett PH *et al*. Increasing prevalence of Type II diabetes in American Indian children. *Diabetologia* 1998; **41**:904–10.
17. Acton KJ, Rios BN, Moore K *et al*. Trends in diabetes prevalence among American Indian and Alaska native children, adolescents, and young adults. *Am J Public Health* 2002; **92**:1485–90.
18. Pinhas-Hamiel O, Dolan LM, Daniels SR *et al*. Increased incidence of non-insulin-dependent diabetes mellitus among adolescents. *J Pediatr* 1996; **128**:608–15.
19. Libman IM, LaPorte RE, Becker D *et al*. Was there an epidemic of diabetes in non-white adolescents in Allegheny County, Pennsylvania? *Diabetes Care* 1998; **21**:1278–81.
20. Lipton R, Keenan H, Onyemere KU *et al*. Incidence and onset features of diabetes in African-American and Latino children in Chicago, 1985–1994. *Diabetes Metab Res Rev* 2002; **18**:135–42.
21. Rosenbloom AL, Joe JR, Young RS *et al*. Emerging epidemic of type 2 diabetes in youth. *Diabetes Care* 1999; **22**:345–54.
22. American Diabetes Association. Type 2 diabetes in children and adolescents. *Diabetes Care* 2000; **23**:381–9.
23. Harris MI, Flegal KM, Cowie CC *et al*. Prevalence of diabetes, impaired fasting glucose, and impaired glucose tolerance in U.S. adults. The Third National Health and Nutrition Examination Survey, 1988–1994. *Diabetes Care* 1998; **21**:518–24.
24. Fagot-Campagna A, Pettitt DJ, Engelgau MM *et al*. Type 2 diabetes among North American children and adolescents: an epidemiologic review and a public health perspective. *J Pediatr* 2000; **136**:664–72.
25. Ferrara A, Imperatore G, Quesenberry CP *et al*. Characteristics and quality of health care of type 1 (T1DM) and type 2 (T2DM) diabetic youths: the Northern California Kaiser Permanente (NCKP) diabetes registry. *Diabetes Care* 2001; **24**:1144–50.
26. Krakoff J, Lindsay RS, Looker HC *et al*. Incidence of retinopathy and nephropathy in youth-onset compared with adult-onset type 2 diabetes. *Diabetes Care* 2003; **26**:76–81.
27. Dean H, Flett B. Natural history of type 2 diabetes diagnosed in childhood: long term follow-up in young adult years. *Diabetes* 2002; **51**:99.
28. Saaddine JB, Engelgau MM, Beckles GL *et al*. A diabetes report card for the United States: quality of care in the 1990s. *Ann Intern Med* 2002; **136**:565–74.
29. McCance DR, Pettitt DJ, Hanson RL *et al*. Birth weight and non-insulin dependent diabetes: thrifty genotype, thrifty phenotype, or surviving small baby genotype? *BMJ* 1994; **308**:942–5.
30. Boloker J, Gertz SJ, Simmons RA. Gestational diabetes leads to the development of diabetes in adulthood in the rat. *Diabetes* 2002; **51**:1499–1506.
31. Dabelea D, Hanson RL, Lindsay RS *et al*. Intrauterine exposure to diabetes conveys risks for type 2 diabetes and obesity: a study of discordant sibships. *Diabetes* 2000; **49**:2208–11.

32. Yajnik CS, Fall CH, Vaidya U *et al.* Fetal growth and glucose and insulin metabolism in four-year-old Indian children. *Diabet Med* 1995; **12**:330–6.
33. Law CM, Gordon GS, Shiell AW *et al.* Thinness at birth and glucose tolerance in seven-year-old children. *Diabet Med* 1995; **12**:24–9.
34. Clausen JO, Borch-Johnsen K, Pedersen O. Relation between birth weight and the insulin sensitivity index in a population sample of 331 young, healthy Caucasians. *Am J Epidemiol* 1997; **146**:23–31.
35. Hales CN, Barker DJ. Type 2 (non-insulin-dependent) diabetes mellitus: the thrifty phenotype hypothesis. *Diabetologia* 1992; **35**:595–601.
36. Poulsen P, Vaag AA, Kyvik KO *et al.* Low birth weight is associated with NIDDM in discordant monozygotic and dizygotic twin pairs. *Diabetologia* 1997; **40**: 439–46.
37. Hattersley AT, Beards F, Ballantyne E *et al.* Mutations in the glucokinase gene of the fetus result in reduced birth weight. *Nat Genet* 1998; **19**:268–70.
38. Dunger DB, Ong KK, Huxtable SJ *et al.* Association of the INS VNTR with size at birth. ALSPAC Study Team. Avon Longitudinal Study of Pregnancy and Childhood. *Nat Genet* 1998; **19**:98–100.
39. Young TK, Martens PJ, Taback SP *et al.* Type 2 diabetes mellitus in children: prenatal and early infancy risk factors among native Canadians. *Arch Pediatr Adolesc Med* 2002; **156**:651–55.
40. Pettitt DJ, Forman MR, Hanson RL *et al.* Breastfeeding and incidence of non-insulin-dependent diabetes mellitus in Pima Indians. *Lancet* 1997; **350**:166–8.
41. Gillman MW, Rifas-Shiman SL, Camargo CA Jr *et al.* Risk of overweight among adolescents who were breastfed as infants. *JAMA* 2001; **285**:2461–7.
42. von Kries R, Koletzko B, Sauerwald T *et al.* Breast feeding and obesity: cross sectional study. *BMJ* 1999; **319**:147–50.
43. Beck LF, Morrow B, Lipscomb LE *et al.* Prevalence of selected maternal behaviors and experiences, Pregnancy Risk Assessment Monitoring System (PRAMS), 1999. *MMWR CDC Surveill Summ* 2002; **51**:1–27.
44. Ogden CL, Flegal KM, Carroll MD *et al.* Prevalence and trends in overweight among US children and adolescents, 1999–2000. *JAMA* 2002; **288**:1728–32.
45. Troiano RP, Briefel RR, Carroll MD *et al.* Energy and fat intakes of children and adolescents in the United States: data from the national health and nutrition examination surveys. *Am J Clin Nutr* 2000; **72**:1343–53S.
46. Cavadini C, Siega-Riz AM, Popkin BM. US adolescent food intake trends from 1965–1996. *Arch Dis Child* 2000; **83**:18–24.
47. Foster-Powell K, Miller JB. International tables of glycemic index. *Am J Clin Nutr* 1995; **62**:871–90S.
48. Salmeron J, Ascherio A, Rimm EB *et al.* Dietary fiber, glycemic load, and risk of NIDDM in men. *Diabetes Care* 1997; **20**:545–50.
49. Salmeron J, Manson JE, Stampfer MJ *et al.* Dietary fiber, glycemic load, and risk of non-insulin-dependent diabetes mellitus in women. *JAMA* 1997; **277**:472–7.
50. Pan XR, Li GW, Hu YH *et al.* Effects of diet and exercise in preventing NIDDM in people with impaired glucose tolerance. The Da Qing IGT and Diabetes Study. *Diabetes Care* 1997; **20**:537–44.
51. Helmrich SP, Ragland DR, Leung RW *et al.* Physical activity and reduced occurrence of non-insulin-dependent diabetes mellitus. *N Engl J Med* 1991; **325**:147–52.

52. Manson JE, Rimm EB, Stampfer MJ *et al*. Physical activity and incidence of non-insulin-dependent diabetes mellitus in women. *Lancet* 1991; **338**:774–8.
53. Manson JE, Nathan DM, Krolewski AS *et al*. A prospective study of exercise and incidence of diabetes among US male physicians. *JAMA* 1992; **268**:63–7.
54. Harding AH, Williams DE, Hennings SH *et al*. Is the association between dietary fat intake and insulin resistance modified by physical activity? *Metabolism* 2001; **50**:1186–92.
55. Regensteiner JG, Shetterly SM, Mayer EJ *et al*. Relationship between habitual physical activity and insulin area among individuals with impaired glucose tolerance. The San Luis Valley Diabetes Study. *Diabetes Care* 1995; **18**:490–7.
56. Grunbaum JA, Kann L, Kinchen SA *et al*. Youth risk behavior surveillance – United States, 2001. *MMWR Surveill Summ* 2002; **51**:1–62.
57. Delisle HF, Ekoe JM. Prevalence of non-insulin-dependent diabetes mellitus and impaired glucose tolerance in two Algonquin communities in Quebec. *CMAJ* 1993; **148**:41–7.
58. Tuomilehto J, Lindstrom J, Eriksson JG *et al*. Prevention of type 2 diabetes mellitus by changes in lifestyle among subjects with impaired glucose tolerance. *N Engl J Med* 2001; **344**:1343–50.
59. Knowler WC, Barrett-Connor E, Fowler SE *et al*. Reduction in the incidence of type 2 diabetes with lifestyle intervention or metformin. *N Engl J Med* 2002; **346**:393–403.
60. Dietz WH, Gortmaker SL. Preventing obesity in children and adolescents. *Annu Rev Public Health* 2001; **22**:337–53.

chapter 4

Type 2 diabetes in children and adolescents in Asia

Kaichi Kida

Introduction

Type 2 diabetes, the predominant type of diabetes in adults, was previously thought to seldom develop in children and adolescents. It is, however, rapidly emerging not only in children and adolescents of particular high-risk ethnic groups but also in Caucasians in parallel with a change of lifestyle in recent decades. Furthermore, type 2 diabetes is now the major type of diabetes in children and adolescents in some high-risk ethnic groups.[1–9] In Asian countries, lifestyles of children and adolescents, as well as those of adults, have changed rapidly, resulting in less physical activity and more fat intake. Consequently, obesity, which is a major risk factor for type 2 diabetes, has steeply increased in children and adolescents.[10,11] The threshold of body mass index (BMI) for the risks of cardiovascular diseases and type 2 diabetes (which are based on insulin resistance) is lower in Asian populations than Caucasian populations, suggesting a genetic predisposition to insulin resistance in Asian populations.[12,13] Loading of these environmental and genetic risk factors for type 2 diabetes in Asian populations is reflected both by the high frequency of childhood and adolescent type 2 diabetes and by its rapid increase in Asian populations, shown by some population-based and hospital-based studies.

Chronic complications develop in children and adolescents with type 2 diabetes as or more quickly than in those with type 1 diabetes. Therefore, an intensive intervention program to promote healthy lifestyles in childhood and adolescence is needed to reduce the risk for type 2 diabetes and thus prevent its chronic complications, particularly in high-risk Asian populations.

Epidemiology

Type 2 diabetes similar to that found in Native Canadian, Native American, African-American and Mexican-American populations[1-7] is emerging in children and adolescents in Asian populations. There is only a limited amount of data on the epidemiology of type 2 diabetes in children and adolescents in Asia, which are based on population studies in Japan and Taiwan. In Japan, all schoolchildren aged 6–15 years have been screened for diabetes by a urine test once a year as determined by a school health law passed in 1993. In some places in Japan, including Tokyo and Yokohama, the diabetes screening program for schoolchildren was launched by their local governments in the 1970s and 1980s. The first morning urine taken at home is examined for glycosuria, followed by a further examination and diagnosis in a medical center for those who are positive for glycosuria. The diagnosis of type 2 diabetes is made by clinical features, an oral glucose tolerance test (OGTT), and measurements of insulin or C-peptide and autoantibodies. All the expenses for the urine screening are covered by the government and those for the further examination and diagnosis by the local government and/or public medical insurance.

The incidence of type 2 diabetes in Japanese schoolchildren aged 6–15 years estimated from results of the diabetes screening program ranges from 4.0 to 7.0 per hundred thousand children per year among different areas in Japan.[8,14,15] (N. Kikuchi, pers. comm.). The incidence of type 2 diabetes in this age group could be somewhat higher than these figures, as it is likely that some cases are missed by urine screening and some cases are found incidentally or clinically before the urine screening. The sensitivity of the urine test for detection of type 2 diabetes is not necessarily high, but almost all cases are thought to be ascertained by this screening as the cases missed in the first screening should be picked up in the screening of the next year. The prevalence of type 2 diabetes in schoolchildren in Osaka is estimated to be $28/100,000(10^5)$ by the capture-mark-recapture method using the diabetes screening program, registries of childhood diabetes and questionnaires to doctors as the three sources of ascertainment.[16]

The incidence and prevalence of type 2 diabetes are 2–4 fold higher than those of type 1 diabetes in Japanese children and adolescents ($1.5/10^5$ per year for incidence and $8.0/10^5$ for prevalence).[17] A rapid increase of type 2 diabetes in schoolchildren has been demonstrated in Tokyo and Yokohama, where the urine diabetes screening program with the urine test for schoolchildren has been conducted since the 1970s and 1980s, i.e. before the nationwide program prescribed by the school health law (Figure 4.1).[8,14–16] The incidence of type 2 diabetes in school-children in Tokyo and Yokohama has increased 3–4 fold over these 25 years – from 1.0–1.5 to $5–7/10^5$ per year. This increase is in parallel with an increase of obesity in the same age group.

In Taiwan, a nationwide diabetes screening program based on urine testing of schoolchildren, similar to the Japanese program, has been in place since 1992. Type 2 diabetes accounts for 60% of diabetes in Taiwanese schoolchildren aged 6–18. The prevalence is estimated to be

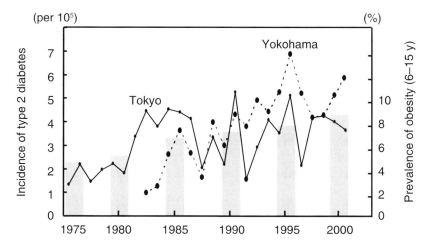

Figure 4.1 *Incidence of type 2 diabetes in Japanese schoolchildren.*

$8.8/10^5$ for boys and $12.2/10^5$ for girls from the results of the diabetes screening program.[18] The Western Pacific Region of International Diabetes Federation (IDF) study to survey the HbA_{1c} of children and adolescents with diabetes was carried out among 96 centers in Australia, China, Indonesia, Japan, Malaysia, the Philippines, Singapore, South Korea, Taiwan and Thailand (IDF WPR Childhood and Adolescence Diabcare 2001 Report), and revealed that type 2 diabetes accounts for 9.8% of diabetes of children and adolescents who have visited the participating diabetes centers during 6 months of the study period.[19] It is likely that the prevalence of type 2 diabetes in children and adolescents in these Western Pacific countries is higher than that shown in the IDF WPR 2001 Report, because a considerable number of children and adolescents with type 2 diabetes are thought to be undiagnosed in some of the regions in the study.

In New Zealand, type 2 diabetes is reported to account for 35% of cases of diabetes diagnosed before the age 30 among Northland Maori registered with the Northland New Zealand Diabetes Service. The majority of young New Zealand Maori patients had type 1 diabetes in studies in the 1980s; thus there is an increasing rate of type 2 diabetes in young New Zealand Maoris.[19] Similarly, a 5-year follow-up study of Australian aborigines revelead that the prevalence of IGT and type 2 diabetes was 1.4% and 1.4%, respectively, at a mean age of 13.3 years and 8.1% and 2.7%, respectively, at a mean age of 18.5 years.[20]

There are a few reports of hospital-based studies indicating increases of childhood and adolescent type 2 diabetes in Asian countries. In a hospital in Bangkok, there were 59 newly diagnosed cases of childhood and adolescent type 2 diabetes for the 10 years from 1987 to 1996 (5.9 cases/year), whereas the number of cases for the 3 years from 1997 to 1999 increased to 39 (13 cases/year).[21] In Singapore, the number of cases of childhood and adolescent type 2 diabetes increased by more than five times over a recent 3-year period in the two biggest diabetes centers for children and adolescents.[22] In the Middle East, as well, there is a report of 5 cases of type 2 diabetes out of 40 cases of diabetes in children and adolescents aged 0–18 years diagnosed in a hospital in the United Arab Emirates during the period 1990–1998.[23] It is thus evident that type 2 diabetes is rapidly emerging in children and adolescents and accounts for a considerable proportion of cases of diabetes in this age group in many parts of Asia.

Clinical features

In Japan and Taiwan, most of the new cases of childhood and adolescent type 2 diabetes are found by the diabetes screening program for school-children before clinical symptoms of the diabetes manifest. In other countries in Asia, most of the cases are found during evaluation of obesity or of symptoms of diabetes such as emaciation, fatigue, polyuria or polydipsia or, incidentally, by examinations for other illnesses. It should be noted that a few percent of children and adolescents with type 2 diabetes have an episode of ketoacidosis at onset of the disease or after-wards (IDF WPR Childhood and Adolescence Diabcare 2001 Report). In Japan, it is reported that some adolescents or young adults with mild type 2 diabetes present with a severe ketosis after drinking a large amount of soft drinks for several days to several weeks. This is called 'soft-drink ketosis' and the relatively low capacity of insulin secretion of Japanese people may make them more prone to this condition.[24]

Type 2 diabetes rarely develops before the age of 5 years and usually begins to develop a few years before puberty followed by a linear increase thereafter.[14,15] The distribution curve of the age of onset in boys is 1.5 years later than in girls, as is puberty, which suggests that changes in insulin sensitivity associated with puberty might be involved in the development of type 2 diabetes. There is almost no significant gender difference in the incidence or prevalence of type 2 diabetes in Japanese children and adoles-cents (M:F = 44:57 in Tokyo and M:F = 49:51 in Yokohama). Similarly, the gender ratio of childhood and adolescent type 2 diabetes registered for the IDF WPR 2001 Report in nine Asian countries excluding Japan is M:F = 48:52. These ratios are different from the female dominance reported in children and adolescents with type 2 diabetes in Native Americans, Native Canadians and Africans.[1-7] In Taiwan, however, female dominance in the incidence of type 2 diabetes in schoolchildren is demonstrated by results in that country's diabetes screening program (M:F = 8.8:12.2).[18]

A strong family history is characteristic of childhood and adolescent type 2 diabetes as it is of adult type 2 diabetes. The prevalence of type 2 diabetes in their parent(s) at diagnosis is 36%,[14] which is far higher than that in the general population of the same age group, and this familial predisposition of type 2 diabetes is comparable to that of type 1 diabetes in the Japanese.[25]

Obesity is one of the characteristic features of childhood and adolescent type 2 diabetes. Obesity is found in 75–85% of Japanese children and adolescents with type 2 diabetes, half of whom manifest only mild obesity (less than 30% in percent overweight for the standard weight).[8,14,15] (N. Kikuchi, pers. comm.) It is thus only 25–30% of children and adolescents with type 2 diabetes who present with severe obesity (50% or more in percent overweight). Similarly, in the IDF WPR 2001 Report, 32% of children and adolescents with type 2 diabetes present with severe obesity equivalent to a BMI of 30 or more in adults whereas 35% and 33% of them had only mild obesity equivalent to adult BMI of 25–30 and normal body weight, respectively. Less frequent association of obesity with type 2 diabetes in Asian populations than in other ethnic groups previously reported in adults suggests that relatively insufficient secretion of insulin might play a role in the development of type 2 diabetes in Asia. However, it is evident that obesity is also a major risk factor for childhood and adolescent type 2 diabetes in Asia. Acanthosis nigricans, which suggests the presence of insulin resistance, is frequently seen in children and adolescents with type 2 diabetes: 57% in Japan (IDF WPR 2001 Report), 85% in Singapore[22] and 71.4% in Thailand.[21] As expected, the acanthosis nigricans is more prevalent in obese children and adolescents with type 2 diabetes than in those without obesity (69% vs 19%) in Japan (IDF WPR 2001 Report), which indicates that relative insufficiency of insulin secretion is predominantly involved in the development of non-obese type 2 diabetes in children and adolescents.

The natural course of type 2 diabetes in children and adolescents seems to be the same as that in adults, and the eye and kidney complications develop in childhood and adolescence-onset type 2 diabetes as fast as or even faster than in type 1 diabetes of the same age group.[26–28] Particularly, microalbuminuria is reported to be present more frequently in young patients with type 2 diabetes than in those with type 1 diabetes (see Chapter 9; IDF WPR 2001 Report; and Ref. 28).

Insulin resistance

The lifestyle of children and adolescents as well as that of adults has been rapidly modernized or westernized, causing a steep increase in obesity in most Asian countries. In Japan, energy intake per capita per day has not changed or even slightly decreased but the energy taken from fat, particularly animal fat, has increased by 2.5 times over the last 30 years.[10] Physical activity of Japanese children and adolescents significantly decreased; 74% of schoolchildren had their physical activity monitored on a certain day in 1981 but this had decreased to 52% in 1992, according to a school health survey.[29] The linear increase of obesity in Japanese schoolchildren, by 2.5 times over the past 30 years, exactly mirrors the modernization or westernization of lifestyle as seen in changes of eating habits and physical activity[10] (Figure 4.2). Similar increasing trends of obesity in parallel with modernization or westernization of lifestyle are seen in children and adolescents in other Asian countries. According to WHO, 6.2 million out of an estimated 22 million children defined as obese in the world are in Southeast Asia and Western Pacific regions.[11]

Obesity is a major risk factor for the development of insulin resistance leading to type 2 diabetes in children and adolescents as it is in adults. In Japanese children and adolescents with obesity, increased insulin secretion and deteriorated glucose tolerance are demonstrated by OGTT, suggesting the development of insulin resistance in parallel with a degree of obesity ($r = 0.52$, $P = 0.001$ and $r = 0.32$, $P = 0.01$) (Figure 4.3).[30] Insulin resistance associated with obesity is further demonstrated by decreased insulin binding to its receptors ($r = -0.69$, $P = 0.001$) and by the increased insulin resistance index 'HOMA-R' (1.25 in control vs 3.90 in obesity, $P = 0.01$)[30,31] Decreased insulin sensitivity associated with obesity in Japanese children and adolescents is more directly shown by the Minimal model (1.2 in control vs 0.45 in obesity, $P = 0.01$) (Figure 4.4).[32]

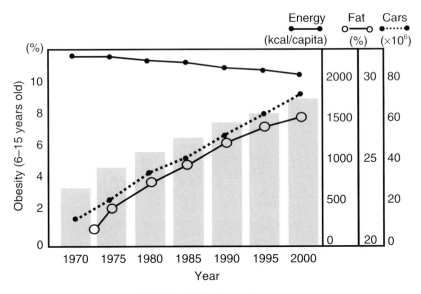

Figure 4.2 *Lifestyle and childhood obesity in Japan.*

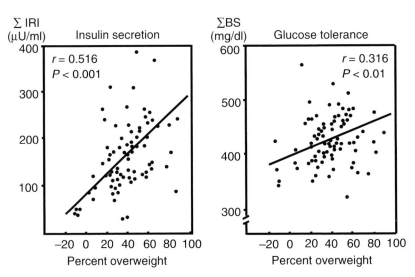

Figure 4.3 *Hyperinsulinemia and glucose intolerance in obese children.*
BS = blood sugar, IRI = insulin resistance index. Source: Kida et al.[30]

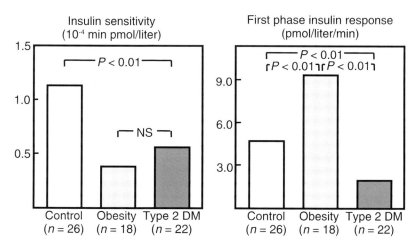

Figure 4.4 *Insulin sensitivity and insulin secretion in children with type 2 diabetes. Source: Kobayashi et al.[32]*

A high prevalence of glucose intolerance is observed in Japanese obese children; impaired glucose tolerance/impaired fasting glucose (IGT/IFG) and type 2 diabetes are found in 15–25% and 4–4.5% of obese children whose percent overweight for the standard weight is 30% or more,[30,33] which is comparable with a recent report on Caucasian, Hispanic and African-American children and adolescents.[34] IGT/IFG associated with obesity in children and adolescents can be reversed by weight reduction, but may lead to type 2 diabetes unless properly treated. In the follow-up studies in Japan, 30% of children and adolescents with IGT/IFG develop type 2 diabetes in 3 years.[35] These findings indicate that insulin resistance associated with obesity is a major risk factor for the development of type 2 diabetes in children and adolescents. It should be noted, however, that the magnitude of insulin resistance is not so different between children with simple obesity and obese children with type 2 diabetes as between normal and obese children. The HOMA-R is 3.9 in simple obesity and 4.8 in obese type 2 diabetes ($P = 0.04$)[31] and there is no difference in insulin sensitivity as estimated by the Minimal model between them.[32] Thus, it is suggested that insufficient secretion of insulin plays an important role in the development of type 2 diabetes in children and adolescents with insulin resistance associated with obesity. In Asian populations, one-fourth of children and adolescents with type 2 diabetes are not obese. The prevalence of acanthosis nigricans is significantly lower (IDR WPR 2001 Report) and both basal and stimulated insulin secretion is significantly less in non-obese children and adolescents with type 2 diabetes than obese ones.[14]

Insufficiency of secretion is considered to be predominantly involved in the development of non-obese type 2 diabetes in children and adolescents. However, it is still likely that insulin resistance is an underlying basis for the development of non-obese type 2 diabetes in children and adolescents since their insulin secretion often has not deteriorated to below the normal ranges and some of them manifest acanthosis nigricans.

Apart from acquired insulin resistance resulting from environmental factors – namely lifestyle – children and adolescents of Asian populations might have genetically lower insulin sensitivity than those of Caucasian populations, as has been shown in Pima Indians and African-Americans.[36–38] This is supported by a finding that the genotype of a mutant β_3-adrenergic receptor gene, one of the candidate genes for insulin resistance, is more prevalent in Asian populations than in Pima Indians.[39–41] Furthermore, the presence of genetic insulin resistance in Japanese children and adolescents is suggested by a finding that serum cholesterol levels are higher in Japanese children and adolescents despite a lower fat intake compared with American children and adolescents.[42]

Treatment

Evidence-based treatment of type 2 diabetes for children and adolescents has not been established but experiences gained in adults can be applied to childhood and adolescent type 2 diabetes. In Asian countries, 31% of children and adolescents with type 2 diabetes are treated by exercise and diet, 41% with an oral hypoglycemic agent, 18% with insulin alone, and 10% with a combination of insulin and hypoglycemic agent (IDF WPR 2001 Report). The oral hypoglycemic agent most commonly used is metformin, the effectiveness and safety of which is proved even in children and adolescents.[43] Metformin is preferably used for obese type 2 diabetes and insulin secretagogues, including sulfonylureas and nateglinide, for non-obese type 2 diabetes. With regard to insulin therapy, 45% of children and adolescents with type 2 diabetes have never been on insulin whereas only 25% of patients are currently on insulin (IDF WPR 2001 Report), which indicates that some of them are able to revert to oral hypoglycemic agents or even to exercise and diet if glucose toxicity is eliminated by strict metabolic control with insulin.

The average metabolic control is better in type 2 diabetes than in type 1 diabetes in Asian patients, but the follow-up studies have shown that chronic complications of retinopathy and nephropathy develop in children and adolescents with type 2 diabetes as fast as or even faster than in those with type 1 diabetes.[26–28] The lack of symptoms in type 2 diabetes often leads to poor compliance or a drop-out from the treatment; 20% of 126 patients have dropped out from treatment in 8 years of follow-up period.[44] A team approach, including pediatric nurse practitioners, is needed for children and adolescents with type 2 diabetes to achieve a good metabolic control and psychosocial well-being.[45] In addition, early detection of type 2 diabetes by screening for children and adolescents with a risk of type 2 diabetes should be carried out to avoid the development of complications, particularly in the high-risk ethnic groups in Asia.[46]

Furthermore, lifestyle intervention with appropriate nutrition and exercise should be a strategy for primary prevention of type 2 diabetes in children and adolescents. Some local governments in Japan run a school-based health promotion program to screen schoolchildren for obesity, dyslipidemia and hypertension and give health education by school nurses, school dieticians and school doctors to children with any of these risks. The results indicate that 50% of schoolchildren with obesity have successfully achieved weight reduction (Figure 4.5).[10] It is similarly reported from Singapore that the percentage of obese children in primary schools has fallen from 12.4% to 10.3% over a 4-year period as a result of the Trim and Fit Program introduced from 1992.[47] There is urgent need to establish a healthy lifestyle through a

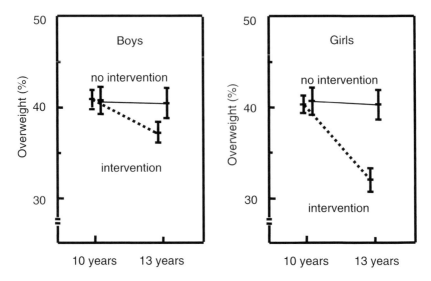

Figure 4.5 *Effect of school-based intervention on childhood and adolescent obesity.*

primary intervention for children and adolescents in order to stop the increasing trend of type 2 diabetes in the world, particularly in Asian countries where the increase is expected to be most significant in the next 20 years.

References

1. Rosenbloom AL, Young RS, Joe JR, Winter WE. Emerging epidemic of type 2 diabetes in youth. *Diabetes Care* 1999; **22**:345–54.
2. Fagot-Campagna A, Pettitt DJ, Engelgau MM *et al*. Type 2 diabetes among North American children and adolescents: epidemiologic review and a public health perspective. *J Pediatr* 2000; **136**:664–72.
3. Dabelea D, Hanson RL, Bennett PH, Roumain J, Knowler WC, Pettitt DJ. Increasing prevalence of type II diabetes in American Indian children. *Diabetologia* 1998; **41**:904–10.
4. Blanchard JF, Dean H, Anderson K, Wajda A, Ludwig S, Depew N. Incidence and prevalence of diabetes in children aged 9–14 years in Manitoba, Canada, 1985–1993. *Diabetes Care* 1997; **20**:512–15.

5. Neufeld ND, Chen Y-DI, Raffel LJ, Vadheim CM, Landon C. Early presentation of type 2 diabetes in Mexican-American youth. *Diabetes Care* 1998; **21**:80–6.
6. Pinhas-Hamiel O, Dolan LM, Daniels SR, Standiford D, Khoury PR, Zeitler P. Increased incidence of non-insulin-dependent diabetes among adolescents. *J Pediatr* 1996; **128**:608–15.
7. Scott CR, Smith JM, Cradock MM, Pihoker C. Characteristics of youth-onset noninsulin-dependent diabetes mellitus at diagnosis. *Pediatrics* 1997; **100**:84–91.
8. Kitagawa T, Owada M, Urakami T, Yamauchi K. Increased incidence of non-insulin dependent diabetes mellitus among Japanese school children correlates with an increased intake of animal protein and fat. *Clin Pediatr* 1998; **37**:111–16.
9. Drake AJ, Smith A, Betts PR, Crowne EC, Shield JP. Type 2 diabetes in obese white childen. *Arch Dis Child* 2002; **86**:207–8.
10. Kida K, Ito T, Yang SW, Tanphaichitr V. Effect of Western diet on risk factors of chronic diseases in Asia. In: Bendich A, Deckelbaum RJ (eds), *Preventive Nutrition*, 2nd edn. New Jersey: Humana Press, 2000:435–46.
11. WHO. World Health Report. Life in the 21st century. Geneva: WHO, 1998: 132.
12. WHO. Obesity. Preventing and managing the global epidemic. Report of a WHO consultation on obesity. Global prevalence and secular trend in obesity. Geneva: WHO, 1997.
13. Tokunaga K, Matsuzawa Y, Kotani K. Ideal body estimated from the body mass index with the lowest morbidity. *Int J Obs* 1991; **15**:1–5.
14. Owada M, Nitadori Y, Urakami T. Studies on characteristics and prognosis of childhood onset type 2 diabetes – screening for school children in Tokyo for 26 years. In: *Diabetology* [in Japanese]. Tokyo: Shindan-to-Chiryousha, 2002: 53–63.
15. Kikuchi N, Shiga K, Tokuhiro E. Epidemiology of childhood onset NIDDM [in Japanese]. *Clin Endocrinol (Tokyo)* 1997; **45**:823–27.
16. Kadoya S, Kawamura T, Kimura Y, Inada H, Ishiki G, Niihira S. Epidemiological study on prevalence of NIDDM of school children in Osaka. *J Jap Diab Soc* 1999; **42**(suppl 1):S236.
17. Kida K, Mimura G, Ito T, Murakami K, Ashkenazi I, Laron Z, Data Committee for Childhood Diabetes of the Japan Diabetes Society (JDS). Incidence of type 1 diabetes mellitus in children aged 0–14 in Japan, 1986–1990, including an analysis for seasonality of onset and month of birth: JDS study. *Diabet Med* 2000; **17**:59–63.
18. Chuang LM, Wei JN, Sung FC *et al.* Incidence and prevalence of childhood diabetes in Taiwan experience with nationwide mass screening. *Diab Res Clin Prac* 2002; **56**(suppl 1):S16.
19. McGrath NM, Parker GN, Dawson P. Early presentation of type 2 diabetes mellitus in young New Zealand Maori. *Diab Res Clin Prac* 1999; **43**:205–9.
20. Braun B, Zimmermann MB, Kretcher N, Spargo RM, Smith RM, Gracey M. Risk factors for diabetes and cardiovascular disease in young Australian aborigines. *Diabetes Care* 1996; **19**:472–9.
21. Likitmaskul S, Tuchinda C, Punnakanta L, Kiattisakthavee P, Chaichanwattanakul K, Angsusingha K. An increase of type 2 diabetes in Thai children and adolescents in Thailand. *J Pediatr Endocrinol Metab* 2000; **13**(suppl 4):1210.

22. Lee WRW, Yap KPF, Loke KY, Hamidah K, Chia YY, Ang S. Characteristics of childhood onset type 2 diabetes in Asia and Singapore. *J Pediatr Endocrinol Metab* 2000; **13**(suppl 4):1209.
23. Punnose J, Agarwal MM, Khdir AE, Devadas K, Mugamer IT. Childhood and adolescent diabetes mellitus in Arabs residing in the United Arab Emirates. *Diab Res Clin Prac* 2002; **55**:29–33.
24. Yamada K, Nonaka K. Diabetic ketoacidosis in young obese Japanese men. *Diabetes Care* 1996; **19**:671.
25. Ito T, Nakamura K, Umeda E *et al*. Familial predisposition of type 1 diabetes in Japan, a country with low incidence. *J Pediatr Endocrinol Metab* 2001; **14**(suppl 1): 589–95.
26. Takahashi H, Sato Y, Matsui M, Urakami T. Ocular fundus findings and systemic factors by type of childhood diabetes. *J Jap Soc Ophthalmol* 1965; **46**:695–9 [in Japanese].
27. Yokoyama H, Okudaira M, Otani T *et al*. Existence of early-onset NIDDM Japanese demonstrating severe diabetic complications. *Diabetes Care* 1997; **20**:844–7.
28. Yokoyama H, Okudaira M, Otani T *et al*. Higher incidence of diabetic nephropathy in type 2 diabetes than in type 1 diabetes in early-onset diabetes in Japan. *Kidney Int* 2000; **58**:302–11.
29. Jap Ass School Health. Report on surveillance of health of school children [in Japanese]. 1992; 57.
30. Kida K, Watanabe N, Fujisawa Y, Goto Y, Matsuda H. The relationship between glucose tolerance and insulin binding to circulating monocytes in obese children. *Pediatrics* 1982; **70**:633–7.
31. Kida K, Goto Y, Watanabe N *et al*. Insulin binding to circulating monocytes with insulin-dependent and non-insulin dependent diabetes mellitus. *Diab Res Clin Prac* 1988; **4**:161–6.
32. Kobayashi K, Amemiya S, Higashida K *et al*. Pathogenic factors of glucose intolerance in obese Japanese adolescents with type 2 diabetes. *Metabolism* 2000; **48**:186–91.
33. Ohki Y, Kishi M, Ohkawa T, Orimo H, Irie M. Current status of frequently observed type 2 diabetes in Japanese children and adolescents – with reference to obesity. *J Pediatr Endocrinol Metab* 2000; **13**(suppl 4):1210.
34. Sinha R, Fish G, Teague B *et al*. Prevalence of impaired glucose tolerance among children and adolescents with marked obesity. *N Engl J Med* 2002; **346**:802–10.
35. Shiga K, Kikuchi. Development of diabetes in children with glucose intolerance (IGT) found by urine screening at school. In: Report of Health and Welfare Science 1999 – Study on causes, treatments and preventions of childhood diabetes and life-style related diseases. *Jap Ministry Health, Welfare and Labor. 2000*; 42–3.
36. Pettitt DJ, Moll PP, Knowler WC *et al*. Insulinemia in children at low and high risk of NIDDM. *Diabetes Care* 1993; **16**:608–15.
37. Arslanian S, Suprasongsin, Janosky JE. Insulin secretion and sensitivity in black versus white prepubertal healthy children. *J Clin Endocrinol Metab* 1997; **82**:1923–7.
38. Barbara A, Gower TR, Goran MI. Visceral fat, insulin sensitivity, and lipids in prepubertal children. *Diabetes* 1999; **48**:1515–21.

39. Walston J, Silver K, Bogardus C *et al*. Time of onset of non-insulin-dependent diabetes mellitus and genetic variation of the β₃-adrenergic-receptor gene. *N Engl J Med* 1995; **333**:343–7.
40. Yoshida T, Sakane U, Umekawa T. Mutation of β₃-adrenergic-receptor gene and response to treatment of obesity. *Lancet* 1995; **346**:1433–4.
41. Kadowaki H, Yasuda K, Iwamoto K *et al*. A mutation in the beta 3-adrenergic receptor gene is associated with obesity and hyperinsulinemia in Japanese subjects. *Biochem Biophys Res Commun* 1995; **215**:555–560.
42. Couch SC, Cross AT, Kida K *et al*. Rapid westernization of children's blood cholesterol in 3 countries: evidence for nutrient–gene interaction. *Am J Clin Nutr* 2000; **72**:1266–72s.
43. Jones KL, Arslanian S, Peterokova VA, Park JS, Tomlinson MJ. Effect of metformin in pediatric patients with type 2 diabetes: a randomized controlled trial. *Diabetes Care* 2002; **25**:89–94.
44. Kikuchi N. Drop-out from treatment in young-onset type 2 diabetes. In: Report of Health and Welfare Science 2000 – study on causes, treatments and preventions of childhood diabetes and life-style related diseases. Jap Ministry Health, Welfare and Labor. 2001; 62.
45. Phillips M, Givens C, Schreiner B. Impact of a multidisciplinary education for children and adolescents with type 2 diabetes. *Diabetes Educ* 2002; **28**:400–2.
46. American Diabetes Association. Consensus statement: type 2 diabetes in children and adolescents. *Diabetes Care* 2000; **23**:381–9.
47. Epidemiology and Disease Control Department, Ministry of Health. National Health Survey. Singapore, 1998.

Acknowledgement

The author is very grateful to Dr. Misao Owada (Associate Professor, Department of Pediatrics, Nihon University Hospital, Tokyo, Japan) and Dr. Nobuyuki Kikuchi, Lecturer, Department of Pediatrics, Yokohama City University Medical Center, Yokohama, Japan) who provided important data for this chapter.

chapter 5

Childhood and adolescent obesity

Louise A Baur and Elizabeth Denney-Wilson

Introduction

Childhood obesity is one of the most serious public health problems facing the developed and, increasingly, the developing world.[1,2] The obesity epidemic is not simply a result of energy imbalance, but rather a consequence of the complex interactions among biological, economic, and social factors. The prevalence of obesity is increasing in children of all ages. Obese children suffer from a host of co-morbidities, some of which are immediately apparent, while others act as warning signs of future disease. Although primary prevention is the most effective strategy in curbing the epidemic, treatment of those children who are currently obese is needed to improve both their immediate and long-term health outcomes.

How is obesity defined in children and adolescents?

Ideally, the definition of overweight and obesity in children should be accurate, easy to perform and equate to health risk. Body mass index (BMI), calculated by dividing weight in kilograms by height in metres squared, is a simple, low-cost measure of body fatness in both adults and children.[3] In adults, the BMI cut-points of 25 kg/m^2 and 30 kg/m^2 are used to define overweight and obesity, respectively, and relate to the point at which health risks rise steeply.[2] Among children, however, there is insufficient evidence to provide an absolute definition of health-related overweight.

Recently, an expert committee convened by the International Obesity TaskForce (IOTF) recommended that BMI, based on centile curves that at age 18 pass through the adult cut-points of 25 kg/m² and 30 kg/m², be used to define overweight and obesity among children and adolescents.[3] Subsequently, Cole and his colleagues developed a table of age- and sex-specific cut-points that can be used particularly in epidemiological research to classify overweight and obesity.[4] Use of this definition allows international comparison of trends in overweight and obesity (see below). In clinical practice, BMI-for-age charts, such as those developed by the Centers for Disease Control and Prevention (CDC) in the United States (see Figures 2.3 and 2.4 on pages 23 and 24) and elsewhere, can be used to chart an individual's BMI and monitor changes.[5] However, the decision about which specific centile lines denote overweight and obesity remains arbitrary.

Abdominal or visceral fat is strongly linked to the co-morbidities of obesity. Waist circumference, even in childhood and adolescence, is strongly correlated with abdominal fat as well as markers for co-morbidities such as adverse lipid and glucose profiles and hypertension.[6] There are no internationally accepted criteria for high- or low-risk waist circumference in children and adolescents.

In defining obesity a further consideration is that racial and ethnic variations exist in the biological response to excess adiposity. For example, Asian adults have a higher percentage body fat for a given BMI than do whites.[7] Studies in the United States have found that African-American, Mexican American and Mohawk Indian children carry more abdominal fat than white children.[8] Acknowledgment of these differences may require the development of ethnic- or race-specific definitions or criteria for obesity. These differences may be important in the primary prevention and management of overweight among racial and ethnic groups.

What is the prevalence of obesity among children and adolescents?

Initially described in Western countries, the obesity epidemic among children has spread throughout the world, with some countries in economic transition such as Uzbekistan, Peru and Nigeria reporting prevalence rates higher than that in the United States.[1] Of further concern is that not only is the prevalence of obesity increasing but the severity of overweight is greater than in the past.[9]

Table 5.1 provides estimates of the prevalence of obesity among children in selected countries, using the IOTF definitions of overweight and obesity. The prevalence of overweight and obesity among children in the United States, Australia, and England is increasing among both boys and girls.[10–12] The prevalence of overweight and obesity in Hong Kong and Singapore is similar to that found a decade earlier in the United States, Australia, and England.[4] In urban areas of China, the prevalence of overweight among children has doubled, from 14.6% in 1989 to 28.9% in 1997, while over the same period, the prevalence of obesity has increased almost 10-fold, from 1.5% to 12.6%.[13] Studies from many other countries, including Belgium, Egypt, Taiwan, Morocco, Finland, and Spain, using different definitions of obesity, have also reported increases in the prevalence of overweight and obesity among children and adolescents.[14]

Sociodemographic differences in the prevalence of obesity

Recent data from the United States indicate sociodemographic differences in the prevalence of obesity among Hispanic (21.8%), African-American (21.5%) and white children (12.3%), with the sharpest increases occurring among African-American and Hispanic children.[15] An inverse social gradient between overweight and socioeconomic groups among both boys and girls has also been shown in Germany.[16]

Among countries in economic transition, however, the association between overweight prevalence and socioeconomic group is reversed.

Table 5.1 Prevalence of overweight and obesity in selected countries, using the IOTF[a] definition

Country	Year of survey	Percent of boys overweight and obese	Percent of boys obese	Percent of girls overweight or obese	Percent of girls obese	Reference
United States	1976–80	14.9	3.4	15.1	4.3	10
United States	1988–94	22.1	7.0	24.0	8.2	10
Australia	1985	10.7	1.4	11.8	1.2	11
Australia	1995	19.5	4.5	21.1	5.3	11
England	1984	5.4	0.6	9.3	1.3	12
England	1994	9.0	1.7	13.5	2.6	12
Singapore	1993	10.5	1.7	7.0	1.0	4
Hong Kong	1993	11.7	3.1	9.8	1.8	4

[a] IOTF = International Obesity TaskForce.[4]

Studies from different countries, including China and Brazil,[13,17] indicate that children and adolescents from higher socioeconomic groups are more likely to be overweight, the possible causes being a greater abundance of energy-dense food, a less strenuous daily life, and greater access to passive entertainment.

What are the health effects of obesity in children and adolescents?

Obese children and adolescents suffer co-morbidities affecting almost every body system (Table 5.2). Immediate effects include social and psychological problems, while long-term effects include the establishment of risk factors for cardiovascular disease and type 2 diabetes and the development of adult obesity.

Psychosocial

The most common consequences of obesity during childhood and adolescence are psychosocial dysfunction and social isolation.[18,19] Preadolescent children associate overweight body shape silhouettes with poor social functioning, impaired academic success and reduced fitness and health,[20] although there is little evidence to suggest that self-esteem is significantly affected in obese young children.[19,21] As would be expected, this situation changes by the time of adolescence. Cross-sectional studies of teenagers show an inverse relationship between weight and both global self-esteem and body-esteem.[21] Obesity in adolescent girls is significantly related to body dissatisfaction, drive for thinness, and bulimia.[22] Adolescence is a period when there is marked self-awareness of body shape and physical appearance, so that it is not surprising that the pervasive, negative social messages associated with obesity in many societies are particularly important at this stage. Overweight in adolescence may also be associated with later social and economic problems. A large prospective study from the USA has shown that women who are overweight in late adolescence and early

Table 5.2 Potential health problems associated with obesity among children and adolescents

System	Health problems
Psychosocial	Social isolation and discrimination, decreased self-esteem, learning difficulties, body image disorder, bulimia *Medium and long term:* poorer social and economic 'success', bulimia
Respiratory	Obstructive sleep apnoea, asthma
Orthopaedic	Back pain, slipped femoral capital epiphyses, tibia vara, ankle sprains, flat feet
Gastrointestinal	Non-alcoholic steatohepatosis, gastro-oesophageal reflux and gastric emptying disturbances, gallstones
Genitourinary	Polycystic ovary syndrome, menstrual abnormalities
Cardiovascular	Hypertension, adverse lipid profile (low HDL cholesterol, high triglycerides, high LDL cholesterol) *Medium and long term:* increased risk of hypertension and adverse lipid profile in adulthood, increased risk of coronary artery disease in adulthood
Endocrine	Hyperinsulinaemia, insulin resistance, type 2 diabetes mellitus *Medium and long term:* increased risk of type 2 diabetes mellitus in adulthood
Neurological	Pseudotumour cerebri

HDL = high-density lipoprotein; LDL = low-density lipoprotein.

adulthood are more likely, as adults, to have lower family incomes, higher rates of poverty and lower rates of marriage than women with other forms of chronic physical disability but who were not over-weight.[23] These findings are likely to reflect social discrimination against obese people.

Orthopaedic

Orthopaedic complications are also well recognized in obese children. In an international multi-centre study, 63% of children with slipped capital femoral epiphyses had a body weight that was greater than or equal to the 90th centile for age.[24] In this problem, the femoral epiphysis is subjected to the increased stress of weight bearing, with eventual slippage occurring. Obesity has also been shown to be more commonly associated with the development of Blount's disease (tibia vara) in which there is a deformity of the medial portion of the proximal tibial metaphysis. As well as these serious forms of orthopaedic disease, more minor abnormalities are also seen, including an increased susceptibility to ankle sprains, knock knee (genu valgum) and flat, wide feet with increased static and dynamic pressures.[25]

Gastrointestinal/hepatobiliary

Hepatic complications of obesity may be present, particularly non-alcoholic hepatic steatosis, which is characterized by mildly raised levels of serum transaminase activities, insulin resistance and, usually, resolution following weight loss.[26] Hepatic cirrhosis may rarely develop. Obesity is the major cause of gallstones in children without other medical problems. Gastro-esophageal reflux and gastric-emptying disturbances are further complications of childhood obesity and appear to be a consequence of raised intra-abdominal pressure from increased subcutaneous and visceral fat.

Neurological

Idiopathic raised intracranial pressure (pseudotumour cerebri) is a very rare complication of childhood obesity that requires immediate recognition and management. About one-third of child and adolescent patients with pseudotumour cerebri are obese,[27] although the role of obesity and other associated conditions in the pathogenesis of the disorder is unknown.

Respiratory

Asthmatic children who are overweight experience more severe respiratory symptoms than do lean children with asthma and they require more medication and more frequent hospital treatment.[28] Obstructive sleep apnoea may occur in obese children and is usually associated with adeno-tonsillar hypertrophy and insulin resistance.[29] Profound hypoventilation and even sudden death have been reported in severe cases of sleep apnoea associated with obesity.

Features of the metabolic syndrome

Obesity, especially central obesity, in childhood is also associated with risk factors for heart disease and type 2 diabetes. Dyslipidaemia is frequently present, the lipoprotein pattern characterised by raised levels of triglycerides and total and low-density lipoprotein (LDL) cholesterol and reduced levels of high-density lipoprotein (HDL) cholesterol.[30] This is particularly related to the presence of increased intra-abdominal fat. Other features of the metabolic syndrome, such as hypertension, hyperinsulinaemia, and insulin resistance, are also commonly seen in centrally obese children.[31] Blood lipid and lipoprotein concentrations, insulin concentrations, and blood pressure all appear to track from childhood into young adulthood, with obesity at baseline being a significant predictor of these measures in adulthood.[18]

The incidence of type 2 diabetes mellitus among children and adolescents is increasing and is inextricably linked to the prevalence of obesity among young people. For example, Pinhas-Hamiel and colleagues reported a 10-fold increase in the estimated incidence of type 2 diabetes among their adolescent referral population, from 0.7/100,000 per year in 1982 to 7.2/100,000 per year in 1994.[32] Other research in the United States suggests that type 2 diabetes accounts for up to one-half of all new cases of paediatric or adolescent diabetes.[33] In this study all of the newly diagnosed adolescents were obese and had family histories of type 2 diabetes.[33] The early onset and increasing prevalence of this disease could pose a major public health problem as more people develop long-term complications at younger ages.

Long-term morbidity and mortality

The most significant long-term consequence of childhood obesity is its persistence into adulthood, with all the attendant health risks.[30] This is more likely with parental obesity, the presence of obesity in late child-hood or adolescence, or with greater severity of obesity.[34] Overweight in adolescence is also associated with long-term mortality and morbidity, a finding that is independent of adult weight and socioeconomic status.[18] Indeed, several long-term cohort studies have shown relative risk estimates of approximately 1.5 for all-cause mortality and 2.0 for mortality from coronary heart disease for overweight children and adolescents when compared to their leaner peers.[18]

Thus, overweight and obesity in childhood and adolescence are associated with a range of psychosocial and medical complications that are both immediate and long term. This makes effective prevention and management vital.

What are the causes of obesity?

Obesity is a complex disorder and, while there is clear evidence for a genetic component to obesity, an appropriate environment must be present in order for obesity to be expressed. The rapid increase in the prevalence of obesity in the past two decades is due to significant changes in the physical and social environment.

Genetic associations of obesity

Twin, adoption, and family studies have shown that there is a strong genetic basis to the development of obesity. The genetic effects account for 25–40%, or possibly more, of the variance in obesity within a population.[34,35] Obesity is a polygenic disorder, with many genes currently linked, or associated, with a predisposition to excess adiposity.[36] Indeed, loci associated with obesity have been identified on all chromosomes but one (chromosome Y).

Candidate genes

There are increasing numbers of reports of candidate genes that have significant associations with obesity-related phenotypes.[36,37] Genes for which there have been at least four separate reports of positive associations with obesity include leptin receptor, peroxisome proliferative activated receptor-γ, glucocorticoid receptor, β-2- and β-3-adrenergic receptors, tumour necrosis factor, leptin, uncoupling proteins 2 and 3, dopamine receptor D2, insulin, guanine nucleotide binding protein β polypeptide 3 and low-density lipoprotein receptor.[37] Not surprisingly, the range of actions of candidate genes is extremely varied, reflecting the many physiological pathways influencing total body energy balance and fat distribution. Thus, genes influencing appetite and satiety signals, the size of the fat depot, adipocyte differentiation, resting metabolic rate, diet-induced thermogenesis, nutrient partitioning, peripheral insulin action, visceral fat and obesity-related co-morbidities are all subjects of intense investigation.[36,37]

Newly described single-gene mutations causing obesity

Mutations in six separate genes leading to severe early-onset obesity in humans have been identified (Table 5.3). The most frequent reports have been made for the melanocortin-4-receptor gene, which is associated with an autosomal dominant form of inheritance. However, in the vast majority of instances of early-onset obesity, no gene mutation has been identified.

Environmental influences on the development of obesity

Obesity is a complex condition, with genetic, metabolic, behavioural, and environmental factors all contributing to its development. However, the dramatic increase in the prevalence of obesity in the past few decades can only be due to significant changes in lifestyle, affecting both children and adults.

Television, computers and video games

The association between television viewing and obesity in childhood and adolescence has been demonstrated in both cross-sectional and longitudinal studies.[38,39] Of particular interest is the finding in some prospective studies that television viewing is associated with an increased incidence of new cases of obesity, as well as a decrease in remission rates of

Table 5.3 Single-gene mutations associated with early-onset obesity in humans

Gene	Probable heritability	Phenotype	Reference
Leptin	Autosomal recessive	Severe early-onset obesity, hyperphagia, hyperinsulinism, hypogonadism	59
Leptin receptor	Autosomal recessive	Severe early-onset obesity, hyperphagia, short stature, central hypothyroidism	60
Pre-pro-opiomelanocortin gene	Autosomal recessive	Severe early-onset obesity, hyperphagia (α-MSH deficiency), adrenal insufficiency (ACTH deficiency), red hair (α-MSH deficiency)	61
Melanocortin-4-receptor	Autosomal dominant	Severe obesity from infancy; normal reproductive function	62,63
Proprotein convertase subtilisin/kexin type 1		Severe early-onset obesity, abnormal glucose homeostasis, hypogonadotrophic hypogonadism, hypocortisolism, raised concentrations of pro-insulin and POMC, decreased concentrations of insulin	64
Single-minded (*Drosophila*) homolog 1		Early-onset obesity, voracious appetite, decreased cortisol and increased insulin concentrations	65

POMC = pre-pro-opiomelanocortin; MSH = melanocyte-stimulating hormone; ACTH = adrenocorticotrophic hormone.

established obesity.[39] Television viewing appears to be a marker of a vulnerable lifestyle and its association with obesity in children and adolescents may reflect some of the following mechanisms:

- exposure of children to food advertising
- increased snacking of energy-dense foods and drinks while watching television
- decreased opportunities for physical activity
- reinforcement of sedentary behaviour.

Dietary intake

The increased prevalence of obesity in recent decades may have resulted, at least in part, from changes in dietary intake, such as an increase in the consumption of high-fat foods or in sugar-containing drinks,[40,41] although the evidence for a clear effect of diet is not strong. In a 12-month prospective study, early school-age children at high risk for the development of obesity were shown to have gained marginally more weight, and consumed a slightly larger proportion of energy from fat than did children at low risk of obesity.[42] Consumption of soda drinks (soft drinks) at baseline is associated with increased weight gain over the next 19 months in young adolescents.[41] In young children, parental influence on food selection is strong, although the influence of television viewing may be significant. In older children and adolescents, peer influence is also important. Less-desirable meal patterns, such as frequent snacking, also appear to be related to obesity.

Physical activity and sedentary behaviour

In the prospective study of low- and high-risk young children mentioned above, the high-risk group (with higher weight gain) had slightly lower levels of total physical activity than did the low-risk group, suggesting a pattern of physical activity that may predispose the at-risk child to the development of obesity.[42] Sedentary behaviour is not merely the inverse of being physically active – they are different, although inter-linked, behaviours. One of the ways in which television viewing may have its association with obesity in childhood is through the encouragement of sedentary behaviour.[39] There are, however, no clear data linking viewing of interactive videos, computers or other 'small-screen' time with the development of obesity, although they are likely to be significantly associated.

Environmental issues in economies in transition

In developing countries and economies undergoing transition, many of the same factors may be influencing the development of obesity. Dietary changes that have accompanied modernization include an increase in consumption of fat, added sugar and animal products in the diet and a decrease in total cereal intake and fibre.[43] Changes in activity level have also occurred as a result of an increase in household labour-saving devices and a rise in television and motor vehicle ownership.[43]

Thus, the increase in sedentary pursuits such as television viewing, video games and computer use, an increase in the use of motorized transport, a decrease in physical activity and an increase in the consumption of high-fat and energy-dense foods are likely to be the major factors in the epidemic of obesity.[2] The early 21st century in industrialized communities provides an environment that is highly conducive to obesity.

What is the management of child and adolescent overweight and obesity?

A systematic review of the treatment of obesity by Glenny *et al.*[44] showed that published studies have used small sample sizes with varying attrition rates (0–56%), and have measured outcomes almost exclusively in terms of degree of overweight, rather than including broader medical, psychosocial and behavioural outcomes. Thus, the evidence to support effective intervention is limited and may not be generalizable to other clinical settings. Nevertheless, the broad principles of management are well recognized (Table 5.4):

- behavioural modification
- family support

- a developmentally appropriate approach
- sensitivity to cultural attitudes and customs
- dietary change
- increased physical activity
- decreased sedentary behaviour.

Clinical assessment

All obese children and adolescents should initially have a full history and physical examination performed. This includes a sensitive exploration of the implications of obesity for the young person and family and of their motivation for behavioural change. A family history of

Table 5.4 Basic elements of behavioural management of obesity in childhood and adolescence

Clarification of treatment outcomes

Family involvement

Developmentally appropriate approach:
- Pre-adolescent children: focus on parents
- Adolescents: separate sessions for the young person

Long-term dietary change:
- Energy reduction
- Lower-fat food choices
- Reduction in high-sugar foods and drinks
- Avoidance of severe dietary restriction

Increase in physical activity:
- Incidental activity
- Active transport options (walking, cycling)
- Lifestyle activities
- Organized activities

Decrease in sedentary behaviour:
- Television, computer and small-screen use
- Alternatives to motorized transport

obesity and disorders associated with insulin resistance (e.g. type 2 diabetes, hypertension, dyslipidaemia, premature heart disease and obstructive sleep apnoea) should be obtained. And, of particular importance, there should be a detailed exploration of the factors influencing physical activity, sedentary behaviour and dietary intake.

Height and weight should be precisely and accurately measured and BMI calculated as weight (kilogram)/height (meter)^2 and then plotted on a BMI-for-age chart. Waist circumference can be used as a proxy for abdominal obesity.[6,8] No specific cut-points for waist-circumference-for-age exist for categorizing abdominal obesity in children and adolescents, but if the waist circumference of a child or adolescent falls above the acceptable waist circumference cut-points for adults (Table 5.5), then he or she can be readily classified as having abdominal obesity. This imperfect, but practical, approach will, of course, lead to an underestimation of abdominal obesity in paediatric patients.

BMI and waist circumference may be most useful in clinical assessment of the individual patient when measured serially and used to monitor change.

Complications that should be sought on physical examination include hypertension, acanthosis nigricans (thickened pigmented skin typically found on the neck and in skin folds, especially the axilla, indicative of insulin resistance), striae, intertrigo, hepatomegaly (fatty

Table 5.5 Sex-specific waist circumference and risk of metabolic complications associated with obesity in Caucasian adults[a]

Risk of metabolic complications	Waist circumference (cm)	
	Men	Women
Increased	≥94	≥80
Substantially increased	≥102	≥88

[a] Presented in the WHO Report[2] and based upon a study of 4881 adults in the Netherlands.[66] Note that the identification of risk using waist circumference cut-points is population-specific.

liver), and an abnormal gait due to joint problems. Warning signs that may indicate other causes for the obesity (e.g. hypothyroidism, hypercortisolism or Prader–Willi syndrome) include short stature, developmental delay, or the presence of dysmorphic features. Note that it is generally very easy to distinguish exogenous obesity associated with a familial predisposition and a vulnerable lifestyle from other, rare, causes of obesity. Biochemical screening for dyslipidaemia, insulin resistance, glucose intolerance, and liver abnormalities should be undertaken in patients with severe obesity, especially if there is a family history of diseases associated with insulin resistance. A history of sleep apnoea should be sought, but this can be difficult to ascertain on questioning.

Defining treatment outcomes

When treating a child or adolescent with obesity the goals of therapy should be initially clarified (Table 5.6). Markers of a successful outcome of therapy may include an improvement in morbidity (e.g. sleep apnoea, hypertension, insulin resistance, dyslipidaemia), psychosocial functioning,

Table 5.6 Defining weight management outcomes

Improvement in complications or behaviour	Improvement in adiposity
Resolution of medical complications, e.g. sleep apnoea, hypertension, insulin resistance, glucose intolerance, dyslipidaemia.	Weight: slowing in rate of weight gain, weight maintenance, weight loss
Improvement in self-esteem and psychosocial functioning	Waist circumference: decrease
Increase in healthy lifestyle behaviours (related to eating, physical activity)	
Increase in level of fitness or aerobic capacity	
Improvement in family functioning	

healthy lifestyle behaviours, aerobic capacity, or family functioning. With regard to change in weight, amelioration of weight gain, rather than substantial weight loss, may be appropriate. Indeed, in younger children, weight maintenance or a reduced rate of weight gain during a growth spurt may be the most achievable approach; in effect, children may be able to 'grow into' an appropriate weight adjusted for height. A decrease in waist circumference is a useful indicator of reduction in abdominal, as well as subcutaneous, obesity.

Education of the family and, where appropriate, the young person, about the nature of obesity, including the realization that it is a chronic disorder of energy balance, is also important, as the need for long-term changes in behaviour will then be more readily apparent. Small, achievable goals are important, e.g. aiming initially for one walk per week or reducing television viewing by 1 h per day every few weeks.

Family focus

Families influence food and activity habits, and thus effective therapy of obesity must take this into account. Parental involvement in treatment programmes is necessary for weight loss, both in young children and in adolescents. Several studies have shown that long-term maintenance of weight loss (i.e. from 2 to 10 years) can be achieved when the intervention is family-based.[45,46] These results have shown that long-term weight control 'success' in childhood obesity is associated with such factors as the amount of weight the parent loses in the initial phase, the use of reinforcement techniques such as parental praise and a change in eating habits, such as eating meals at home or a moderate reduction in fat intake.[45,46] Such findings imply that altered food patterns within the whole family, as well as support of the child and parental reinforcement of a healthy lifestyle, are important factors in successful outcomes.

A developmentally appropriate approach

There is increasing evidence that treatment of pre-adolescent obesity with the parents as the *exclusive* agents of lifestyle change is superior to a child-centred approach.[47,48] An Israeli study randomized obese children aged 6–11 years and their parents to either an experimental intervention where only the parents attended group sessions (with an emphasis on general parenting skills), or a control intervention where only the children attended group sessions.[47,48] There was a greater reduction in overweight in the experimental group, with children in the control group having higher rates of reported anxiety and of withdrawal from the programme. Thus, when dealing with the obese pre-adolescent child, sessions involving the parent or parents alone, without the child being present, are likely to be the most effective.

A different approach is needed for the adolescent patient. Features of successful interventions in adolescent obesity include the provision of separate sessions for the adolescent patient and the parent, and having a structured, although flexible, programme that encourages sustainable modifications in lifestyle, relationships and attitudes.[49,50] There is also a report of at least short-term success in management of adolescent obesity with a phone- and mail-based behavioural intervention initiated in a primary care setting.[51]

Dietary management

In the past, more prescriptive dietary approaches were used in the treatment of paediatric obesity, but the current approach generally involves education about healthy nutrition and appropriate food choices, including a low-fat diet. There are many metabolic reasons why a high-fat diet may cause problems with regulation of energy balance, as well as evidence from adult studies that a low-fat diet is helpful in promoting weight loss in obese patients.[40] In the management of childhood obesity, a moderate restriction in fat intake in the initial phase of therapy is associated with sustained treatment effects.[46] A low glycaemic index diet has been proposed as useful in the management of childhood obesity but no prospective studies have been performed using this treatment approach.[52]

There is no direct evidence for which dietary modification is most effective for weight management in children and adolescents. Dietary interventions should follow national nutrition guidelines and have an emphasis on lower fat options, more vegetable and fruit intake, healthier snack food choices and, possibly, decreased portion sizes. A reduction in soft drink or fruit juice intake is also important in decreasing total energy intake.[41] Involvement of the entire family in making the change to a sustainable and healthy food intake is vital. This is because changes in shopping and cooking practices, and altered attitudes to snacking and mealtimes, are required. The focus should be on behaviour change, healthier food choices, and a reduction in fat content of foods and in consumption of high-sugar drinks. Avoidance of severe dietary restriction may be an important strategy in helping the development of the child's capacity to self-regulate dietary intake. Restrictive dieting may also interfere with growth in childhood or encourage the development of an eating disorder. Nevertheless, a flexible and individualized diet prescription may be useful in helping a family or young person to make the transition to sustained healthy eating habits.

Physical activity and sedentary behaviour

Epstein *et al.*[53] have shown that participation of children in an exercise programme during treatment for obesity is a predictor of long-term successful weight control. The type of exercise employed (i.e. 'lifestyle' exercise versus programmed aerobic exercise) also appears to be important for sustained weight loss; while both forms of exercise help promote weight loss in the initial phase, the child or adolescent is more likely to continue long term with the 'lifestyle' form of exercise.[53] Families and young people need to be reminded that increased physical activity may best result from a change in incidental activity and not necessarily from organized activities such as school sport. Importantly, children and adolescents should be encouraged to choose activities that they enjoy and which are therefore likely to be more sustainable.

A further controlled study has looked at the effect of targeting inactivity. Epstein's group[54] has shown that 2-year outcome was most successful for children who were placed in a group in which sedentary behaviour was targeted rather than in those children who were in groups where they were encouraged to increase their level of exercise. Thus, limitation of television viewing, video games and computer games may encourage children to choose more active pursuits.[39,54]

Parental involvement is vital if an increase in physical activity or a decrease in sedentary behaviour is to occur. This may include monitoring television use, role-modelling of healthy behaviours, encouragement and providing access to recreation areas or recreational equipment.

Types of interventions

Even in the management of adult obesity there have been few studies looking at the effectiveness of different types of interventions (e.g. group programmes, individual counselling sessions, sessions delivered by different types of health care professional), or interventions delivered in different settings (e.g. primary care, community health centre, tertiary institutions).[55] When dealing with obese children and adolescents, there is some evidence that time-efficient interventions such as group sessions, holiday camps, or mail- and phone-based behavioural interventions do at least as well as individual sessions.[51,56]

Other forms of therapy

The current clinical management of paediatric obesity involves behavioural therapy. There is little information to guide the use of more aggressive treatment approaches such as protein-sparing modified fasts, obesity surgery, or drug therapy in the treatment of paediatric obesity. Experience from adult studies suggests that they need to be used in the context of a behavioural management programme. No pharmacological agents are currently approved for the treatment of paediatric obesity, although therapeutic trials are underway with drugs such as orlistat and sibutramine. Until further randomized controlled trials of such therapies are available, they should only be considered for obese young people who have failed conventional management and have significant complications of their obesity. Such therapies, if used at all, should occur in the context of a behavioural weight management programme and be restricted to specialist centres with expertise in managing morbid obesity.

Obesity prevention

The magnitude of the problem of obesity in most industrialized and industrializing countries means that, to prevent further increases in prevalence, population-level strategies must be applied.[2] Interventions focussing on simply educating individuals and communities about behaviour change have had limited or no success. Instead, there is a need to produce an environment that supports healthy eating and physical activity throughout the community. This requires a commitment from many sectors of society.

A recently published systematic review of interventions for preventing obesity in children concluded that there are 'limited high quality data on the effectiveness of prevention programs'.[57] This may well reflect the methodological and ethical challenges in conducting such studies, often in a sociopolitical environment that is not conducive to change. However, the published studies do highlight the potential of both a reduction in sedentary behaviours and an increase in physical activity in prevention programmes.

The factors promoting the development of child and adolescent obesity may be operating at both a micro-environmental level (i.e. the settings where individuals live, eat, play or go to school) as well as at a macro-environmental level (i.e. the broader sectors that ultimately influence dietary intake and physical activity and which are beyond the ability of an individual to influence).[58] Table 5.7 lists examples of the settings that may be important in influencing the development of obesity. When these are considered, it is apparent that opportunities exist for a range of prevention strategies in a given community. These might include:

- regulation of the nature and amount of food advertising directed at children
- provision of high-quality recreation areas
- regulation of types of food and drink provided in school canteens
- provision of innovative physical education programmes in schools that offer a range of fun and energetic opportunities beyond competitive sports, such as dancing, martial arts and aerobics
- improvement in public transport
- provision of safe cycle paths and safe street lighting in local neighbourhoods

Table 5.7 Examples of micro-environment settings and macro-environment sectors for the prevention of obesity[a]

Micro-environment settings	Macro-environment sectors
Homes	Technology and design (e.g. labour-saving devices, architecture)
Schools	
Community groups (e.g. clubs, churches)	Food production and importing
	Food manufacturing and distribution
Community places (e.g. parks, shopping malls)	Food marketing (e.g. fast food advertising)
Institutions (e.g. boarding schools)	Food catering services
Food retailers (e.g. supermarkets)	Sports and leisure industry (e.g. instructor training programmes)
Food service outlets (e.g. canteens, lunch bars, restaurants)	
Recreation facilities (e.g. pools, gyms)	Urban and rural development (e.g. town planning, local government)
Neighbourhoods (e.g. cycle paths, street safety)	Transport system (e.g. public transportation systems)
Local health care	Health system

[a] Adapted from Swinburn et al.[58]

- support of walk-to-school programmes
- provision of economic incentives for the production and distribution of vegetables and fruit
- development of town planning policies which promote active transport or public transport over motorized transport.

There are few examples of successful multifaceted large-scale interventions to guide obesity prevention. Such interventions will require inter-sectoral and inter-governmental cooperation, supported by adequate resources and significant community ownership.

References

1. Deckelbaum RJ, Williams CL. Childhood obesity: the health issue. *Obes Res* 2001; **Suppl 4**:239–43S.
2. WHO. Obesity: preventing and managing the global epidemic. Report of a WHO consultation on obesity. Geneva: WHO, 1998.
3. Bellizzi MC, Dietz WH. Workshop on childhood obesity: summary of the discussion. *Am J Clin Nutr* 1999; **70**:173–5S.
4. Cole TJ, Bellizzi MC, Flegal KM, Dietz WH. Establishing a standard definition for child overweight and obesity worldwide: international survey. *BMJ* 2000; **320**:1240–3.
5. Kuczmarski RJ, Ogden CL, Grummer-Strawn LM *et al*. CDC growth charts: United States. *Advance Data* 2000; **341**:1–27. Web-site: http://www.cdc.gov/**growthcharts**
6. Maffeis C, Pietrobelli A, Grezzani A *et al*. Waist circumference and cardiovascular risk factors in prepubertal children. *Obes Res* 2001; **9**:179–87.
7. Wang J, Thornton JC, Russell M *et al*. Asians have lower body mass index (BMI) but higher percent body fat than do whites: comparison of anthropometric measurements. *Am J Clin Nutr* 1994; **60**:23–8.
8. Goran MI, Gower BA. Relation between visceral fat and disease risk in children and adolescents. *Am J Clin Nutr* 1999; **70**:149–56S.
9. Troiano RP, Flegal KM. Overweight children and adolescents: description, epidemiology and demographics. *Pediatrics* 1998; **Suppl 2**:497–504.
10. Flegal KM, Ogden CL, Wei R *et al*. Prevalence of overweight in US children: comparison of US growth charts from the Centers for Disease Control and Prevention with other reference values for body mass index. *Am J Clin Nutr* 2001; **73**:1086–93.
11. Magarey AM, Daniels LA, Boulton TJ. Prevalence of overweight and obesity in Australian children and adolescents: reassessment of 1985 and 1995 data against new standard international definitions. *MJA* 2001; **174**:561–4.
12. Chinn S, Rona RJ. Prevalence and trends in overweight and obesity in three cross sectional studies of British Children, 1974–94. *BMJ* 2001; **322**:24–6.
13. Luo J, Hu FB. Time trends of obesity in pre-school children in China from 1989 to 1997. *Int J Obes* 2002; **6**:553–8.
14. www.iotf.org
15. Strauss RS, Pollack HA. Epidemic increase in childhood overweight, 1986–1998. *JAMA* 2001; **286**:2845–8.
16. Langnase K, Mast M, Muller MJ. Social class differences in overweight of prepubertal children in northwest Germany. *Int J Obes* 2002; **26**:566–72.
17. Neutzling MB, Taddei JA, Rodrigues EM, Sigulem DM. Overweight and obesity in Brazilian adolescents. *Int J Obes* 2000; **24**:869–74.
18. Must A, Strauss RS. Risks and consequences of childhood and adolescent obesity. *Int J Obes* 1999; **23**(Suppl 2):S2–11.
19. French SA, Story M, Perry CL. Self-esteem and obesity in children and adolescents: a literature review. *Obes Res* 1995; **3**:479–90.
20. Hill AJ, Silver EK. Fat, friendless and unhealthy: 9 year old children's perception of body shapestereotypes. *Int J Obes* 1995; **19**:423–30.

21. Klesges RC, Haddock CK, Stein RJ *et al*. Relationship between psychosocial functioning and body fat in preschool children: a longitudinal investigation. *J Consult Clin Psychol* 1992; **60**:793–6.

22. Freidman MA, Wilfley DE, Pike KM *et al*. The relationship between weight and psychological functioning among adolescent girls. *Obes Res* 1995; **57**: 57–62.

23. Gortmaker SL, Must A, Perrin JM *et al*. Social and economic consequences of overweight in adolescence and young adulthood. *N Engl J Med* 1993; **329**:1008–12.

24. Loder RT. The demographics of slipped capital femoral epiphysis. An international multicenter study. *Clin Orthop* 1996; **322**:8–27.

25. Dowling AM, Steel JR, Baur LA. Does obesity influence foot structure and plantar pressure patterns in prepubescent children? *Int J Obes* 2001; **25**:845–52.

26. Guzzaloni G, Grugni G, Minocci A *et al*. Liver steatosis in juvenile obesity: correlations with lipid profile, hepatic biochemical parameters and glycemic and insulinemic responses to an oral glucose tolerance test. *Int J Obes* 2000; **24**:772–6.

27. Scott IU, Siatkowski RM, Eneyni M *et al*. Idiopathic intracranial hypertension in children and adolescents. *Am J Ophthalmol* 1997; **124**:253–7.

28. Belmarich PF, Luder E, Kattan M *et al*. Do obese inner-city children with asthma have more symptoms than nonobese children with asthma? *Pediatrics* 2000; **106**:1436–41.

29. de la Eva RC, Baur LA, Donaghue K, Waters KA. Metabolic correlates with obstructive sleep apnea. *J Pediatr* 2002; **140**:654–9.

30. Freedman DS, Dietz WH, Srinivasan SR, Berenson GS. The relation of overweight to cardiovascular risk factors among children and adolescents: The Bogalusa Heart Study. *Pediatrics* 1999; **103**:1175–82.

31. Srinivasan SR, Bao W, Wattigney WA, Berenson GS. Adolescent overweight is associated with adult overweight and multiple cardiovascular risk factors: the Bogalusa heart study. *Metabolism* 1996; **45**:235–40.

32. Pinhas-Hamiel O, Dolan LM, Daniels SR, Standiford D *et al*. Increased incidence of non-insulin-dependent diabetes mellitus among adolescents. *J Pediatr* 1996; **128**:608–15.

33. Fagot-Campagna A, Pettitt DJ, Engelgau MM *et al*. Type 2 diabetes among North American children and adolescents: an epidemiologic review and a public health perspective. *J Pediatr* 2000; **136**:664–72.

34. Whitaker RC, Wright JA, Pepe MS *et al*. Predicting obesity in young adulthood from childhood and parental obesity. *N Engl J Med* 1997; **337**:869–73.

35. Stunkard AJ, Harris JR, Pedersen NL, McClearn GE. The body-mass index of twins who have been reared apart. *N Engl J Med* 1990; **322**:1483–7.

36. Ukkola O, Bouchard C. Clustering of metabolic abnormalities in obese individuals: the role of genetic factors. *Ann Med* 2001; **33**:79–90.

37. Rankinen T, Perusse L, Weisnagel J *et al*. The human obesity map: the 2001 update. *Obes Res* 2002; **10**:196–243.

38. Dietz WH, Gortmaker SL. Do we fatten our children at the television set? Obesity and television viewing in children and adolescents. *Pediatrics* 1985; **75**:807–12.

39. Robinson TN. Television viewing and childhood obesity. *Pediatr Clin North Am* 2001; **48**:1017–25.
40. Astrup A. The role of dietary fat in the prevention and treatment of obesity. Efficacy and safety of low-fat diets. *Int J Obesity* 2001; **25**(Suppl 1):S46–50.
41. Ludwig DS, Peterson KE, Gortmaker SL. Relation between consumption of sugar-sweetened drinks and childhood obesity: a prospective, observational analysis. *Lancet* 2001; **357**:505–8.
42. Eck LH, Klesges RC, Hanson CL, Slawson D. Children at familial risk of obesity: an examination of dietary intake, physical activity and weight status. *Int J Obes* 1992; **16**:71–8.
43. Popkin BM. The nutrition transition and obesity in the developing world. *J Nutr* 2001; **131**:871–3S.
44. Glenny A-M, O'Meara S, Melville A *et al*. The treatment and prevention of obesity: a systematic review of the literature. *Int J Obes* 1997; **21**:715–37.
45. Epstein LH, Valoski A, Wing RR, McCurley J. Ten-year follow-up of behavioural, family-based treatment for obese children. *JAMA* 1990; **264**:2519–23.
46. Nuutinen O, Knip M. Predictors of weight reduction in obese children. *Eur J Clin Nutr* 1992; **46**:785–94.
47. Golan M, Weizman A, Apter A, Fainaru M. Parents as the exclusive agents of change in the treatment of childhood obesity. *Am J Clin Nutr* 1998; **67**:1130–5.
48. Golan M, Fainaru M, Weizman A. Role of behaviour modification in the treatment of childhood obesity with the parents as the exclusive agents of change. *Int J Obes* 1998; **22**:1217–24.
49. Brownell KD, Kelman JH, Stunkard AJ. Treatment of obese children with and without their mothers: changes in weight and blood pressure. *Pediatrics* 1993; **71**:515–23.
50. Mellin LM, Slinkard LA, Irwin CE. Adolescent obesity intervention: validation of the SHAPEDOWN program. *J Am Diet Assoc* 1987; **87**:333–8.
51. Saelens BE, Sallis JF, Wilfley DE *et al*. Behavioral weight control for overweight adolescents initiated in primary care. *Obes Res* 2002; **10**:22–32.
52. Speith LE, Harnish JD, Lenders CM *et al*. A low-glycemic index diet in the treatment of pediatric obesity. *Arch Pediatr Adolesc Med* 2000; **154**:947–51.
53. Epstein LH, Wing RR, Koeske R *et al*. A comparison of lifestyle change and programmed exercise on weight and fitness changes in obese children. *Behav Ther* 1982; **13**:651–65.
54. Epstein LH, Roemmich JN. Reducing sedentary behavior: role in modifying physical activity. *Exerc Sport Sci Rev* 2001; **29**:103–8.
55. Harvey EL, Glenny A-M, Kirk SFL, Summerbell CD. Improving health professionals' management and the organisation of care for overweight and obese people (Cochrane Review). In: *The Cochrane Library, Issue 2*, 1999. Oxford: Update Software.
56. Braet C, van Winckel M, van Leeuwen K. Follow-up results of different treatment programs for obese children. *Acta Paediatr* 1997; **86**:397–402.
57. Campbell K, Waters E, O'Meara S, Summerbell C. Interventions for preventing obesity in children (Cochrane Review). In: *The Cochrane Library, Issue 2*, 2002. Oxford: Update Software.

58. Swinburn B, Egger G, Fezeela R. Dissecting obesogenic environments: the development and application of a framework for identifying and prioritising environmental interventions for obesity. *Prev Med* 1999; **29**:563–70.
59. Montague CT, Farooqi IS, Whitehead JP *et al*. Congenital leptin deficiency is associated with severe early-onset obesity in humans. *Nature* 1997; **387**: 903–8.
60. Clement K, Vaisse C, Lahlou N *et al*. A mutation in the human leptin receptor gene causes obesity and pituitary dysfunction. *Nature* 1998; **392**:398–401.
61. Krude H, Biebermann H, Luck W *et al*. Severe early-onset obesity, adrenal insufficiency and red hair pigmentation caused by POMC mutations in humans. *Nature Genetics* 1988; **19**:155–7.
62. Vaisse C, Clement K, Guy-Grand B, Froguel P. A frameshift mutation in human MC4R is associated with a dominant form of obesity. *Nature Genetics* 1998; **20**:113–14.
63. Yeo GS, Farooqi IS, Aminian S *et al*. A frameshift mutation in MC4R associated with dominantly inherited human obesity. *Nature Genetics* 1998; **20**:111–12.
64. Jackson RS, Creemers JW, Ohagi S *et al*. Obesity and impaired prohormone processing associated with mutations in the human prohormone convertase 1 gene. *Nature Genetics* 1997; **16**:303–6.
65. Holder JL Jr, Butte NF, Zinn AR. Profound obesity associated with a balanced translocation that disrupts the SIM1 gene. *Hum Mol Gen* 2002; **9**:101–8.
66. Han TS, Leer EM, Seidell JC, Lean MEJ. Waist circumference action levels in the identification of cardiovascular risk factors: prevalence study in a random sample. *BMJ* 1995; **311**:1401–5.

chapter 6

Insulin resistance and insulin secretion in childhood and adolescence: their role in type 2 diabetes in youth

Silva A Arslanian

Introduction

Type 2 diabetes mellitus is a complex metabolic disorder of heterogeneous etiology, with social, behavioral, and environmental risk factors unmasking the underlying genetic susceptibility of individuals.[1] Insulin resistance and impaired insulin secretion are the two pathophysiological abnormalities responsible for type 2 diabetes. There is clearly a strong hereditary component to the disease, which is likely to be multigenic in nature.[2] The important role of genetic determinants is well illustrated when differences in the prevalence of type 2 diabetes in various racial/ethnic groups are considered.[3] However, even though genetic susceptibility to type 2 diabetes is important, the escalating prevalence of type 2 diabetes in youth is occurring too quickly to be the result of increased gene frequency and altered genetic pool. Environmental lifestyle factors play an important role. This chapter will review insulin sensitivity and secretion in childhood and discuss the factors responsible for abnormalities in either parameter that may lead to the expression of type 2 diabetes.

Insulin resistance, insulin secretion, and the risk of type 2 diabetes

In its fully manifested phenotype, type 2 diabetes is characterized by insulin resistance, involving both hepatic and peripheral tissues, and relative insulin deficiency. Glucose homeostasis depends on the delicate balance between insulin action in insulin-sensitive tissues and insulin secretion by the pancreatic beta cells. The nature of this balance is such that insulin sensitivity and beta-cell function are inversely and proportionately related in a hyperbolic function so that their product is always a constant, referred to as the glucose disposition index (DI).[4–6] Such a relationship implies that differences in insulin sensitivity must be balanced by reciprocal changes in beta-cell function to maintain glucose tolerance. The DI seems to be a heritable characteristic.[6,7] Those at risk for diabetes have a lower DI, reflecting the inability of the beta cells to compensate for insulin resistance. Thus, insulin resistance alone is not sufficient to cause full-blown hyperglycemia, which will develop only if insulin secretion by the beta cells is inadequate. There has been considerable debate, however, about whether insulin resistance or insulin hyposecretion is the primary or the earliest defect in type 2 diabetes in adults.[8–10] Studies on type 2 diabetes in youth are limited because it has only recently become common as a pediatric condition. In this chapter the hypothesis is put forward that the early abnormality in youth type 2 diabetes is insulin resistance, compounded later by beta-cell failure and insulin deficiency (Figure 6.1). This chapter focuses on insulin sensitivity and secretion during childhood growth and development. Physiological and pathophysiological factors that modulate insulin sensitivity and secretion will be discussed. Finally, although we do not understand all the possible mechanisms responsible for the functional alterations leading to type 2 diabetes in children, the information that is gradually being gathered is summarized. Gaining insight into the pathophysiological alterations responsible for type 2 diabetes in childhood will likely bear on our choices of therapy and on our ability to treat this relentless metabolic disorder.

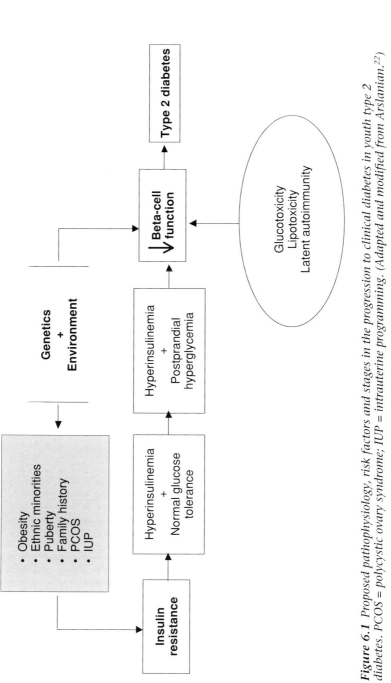

Figure 6.1 *Proposed pathophysiology, risk factors and stages in the progression to clinical diabetes in youth type 2 diabetes. PCOS = polycystic ovary syndrome; IUP = intrauterine programming. (Adapted and modified from Arslanian.[22])*

The fact that a large number of adult patients with DM are 'insulin insensitive' was first demonstrated by Himsworth more than 60 years ago.[11] Since then, it has been recognized that resistance to insulin-stimulated glucose uptake is a characteristic finding in adult patients with type 2 diabetes and impaired glucose tolerance.[12] Cross-sectional and longitudinal studies have been performed in adult populations at high risk for developing type 2 diabetes, such as the Pima Indians, Nauruans (a population of Pacific islanders), and Mexican Americans. These studies demonstrate that hyperinsulinemia and insulin resistance are present in the prediabetic normoglycemic state.[13-18] However, in adults with clinical type 2 diabetes, impaired insulin action and insulin secretory failure are both present.[14,19-21] The failure of beta cells to continue to hypersecrete insulin thus underlies the transition from insulin resistance with compensatory hyperinsulinemia and normoglycemia, to impaired glucose tolerance with mild increases in postprandial glucose concentrations, and then to clinical diabetes with overt fasting hyperglycemia and increased hepatic glucose production (Figure 6.1).[22]

Abnormalities of insulin secretion in adults with type 2 diabetes include reduced or absent first-phase responses to intravenous glucose, delayed and blunted secretory responses to the ingestion of a mixed meal, alterations in the rapid pulses and ultradian oscillations of insulin secretion, and increases in the plasma concentrations of proinsulin-like peptides relative to those of insulin.[6,20,21] Studies of youths with type 2 diabetes are almost nonexistent, but they would most likely mirror adult findings.

To date, there is uniform agreement among the published reports that youth type 2 diabetes occurs in:

1. children who are obese
2. children who are predominantly from minority ethnic populations (African-Americans, Hispanics, etc.), but whites are also affected
3. children who are typically in mid-puberty
4. children who have a strong family history of type 2 diabetes
5. children who have conditions associated with insulin resistance, e.g. polycystic ovary syndrome (PCOS), hypertension, 'syndrome X', acanthosis nigricans.[23-28]

All of these risk factors have in common insulin resistance/hyperinsulinemia initially (Figure 6.1).[22] The rest of this chapter reviews the current state of knowledge with respect to insulin sensitivity and secretion regarding each risk condition.

Obesity, insulin sensitivity, and secretion

Obesity is now the most common nutritional disease of children in the United States. A recent survey, 1999–2000, of 4722 children from birth through to 19 years of age, as part of the National Health and Nutrition Examination Survey (NHANES), shows that the prevalence and severity of obesity continue to escalate.[29] The prevalence of overweight – body mass index (BMI) for age $\geq$ 95th percentile – was approximately 10% for 2–5 year olds and 15% for 6–11 year olds and 12–19 year olds.[29] The prevalence of overweight among 12–19-year-old non-Hispanic blacks (23.6%) and Mexican Americans (23.4%) was significantly higher than among non-Hispanic whites (12.7%). Also, there is a 'global epidemic of obesity' that is a rapidly growing threat to the health of populations in an increasing number of countries.[30,31]

Obesity is a health risk not only in adulthood but also in childhood.[32,33] Cross-sectional and longitudinal studies have shown that obesity and increased abdominal fat distribution are major risk factors in adults for type 2 diabetes in all populations.[34] This risk is imparted through the negative impact of obesity on insulin action.[35,36] The effects of obesity on glucose metabolism are evident early in childhood. Our research has demonstrated that in healthy Caucasian children, total body adiposity accounts for 55% of the variance in insulin sensitivity.[37] This negative impact of obesity on insulin sensitivity is also evident in black children.[38] Obese children have peripheral insulin resistance, with ~40% lower insulin-stimulated glucose metabolism compared with non-obese children.[33] This decrease in insulin-stimulated glucose metabolism involves both glucose oxidation and glucose storage.[33] The insulin resistance of obesity is not limited to glucose metabolism but also involves lipid metabolism. Suppression of lipolysis with insulin is impaired in obese adolescents compared with lean controls.[33] Moreover, the amount of visceral fat in children, lean or obese, black or white, plays an important role in the impaired insulin sensitivity.[39,40]

Despite the presence of insulin resistance, glucose homeostasis remains relatively normal for long periods in obesity. This occurs because of increased insulin secretion to compensate for the lower insulin action. In obese children, fasting and stimulated insulin levels are higher than in non-obese controls.[33,41–43] However, when insulin secretion declines in the face of insulin resistance, glucose homeostasis deteriorates. Data from obese Japanese adolescents demonstrate that the compensatory increase in first-phase insulin response is diminished with the progression to severe type 2 diabetes.[42] Similarly, C-peptide response to a mixed meal (Sustacal) is significantly lower in adolescents with type 2 diabetes than in the matched controls.[44] Thus, even though obesity is a major risk factor for type 2 diabetes, not all obese subjects develop diabetes unless the delicate balance between insulin action and secretion is disturbed.

Race, insulin sensitivity, and secretion

There are convincing epidemiological and clinical research data showing that black children are more hyperinsulinemic/insulin resistant than their white peers.[45–52] In the Bogalusa Heart Study of 377 children, 5–17-year-old black children and adolescents had higher insulin responses during an oral glucose tolerance test (OGTT) than did white children, even after adjusting for ponderal index.[45] Similarly, fasting insulin levels were higher in black 7–11-year-old children compared with whites.[47] These results suggested that insulin sensitivity was lower in blacks but compensated with increased insulin secretion. In our earlier studies of prepubertal healthy children, fasting and first-phase insulin concentrations during a hyperglycemic clamp were significantly higher in blacks than whites.[48] Similarly, in pubertal adolescents, insulin secretion was higher in blacks.[49]

Other investigators, using the tolbutamide-modified frequently sampled intravenous glucose tolerance test (IVGTT) with minimal modeling, demonstrated lower insulin sensitivity and higher acute insulin response in black vs white prepubertal children.[50,51] In addition, the hyperinsulinemia in black children is attributed to lower insulin clearance as manifested in lower ratios of C-peptide to insulin.[46,51] Our recent observations indicate that insulin clearance is ~15% lower in black prepubertal children compared with whites matched for age, BMI, body composition, and abdominal adiposity.[52]

Based on such information, the general agreement is that the hyperinsulinemia in black children is an adaptive mechanism to compensate for the lower insulin sensitivity by increased insulin secretion and decreased insulin clearance. The lower insulin sensitivity in blacks may play a role in the higher rates of type 2 diabetes whether in adults or children. Insulin resistance alone, however, does not cause diabetes. Therefore, in a recent investigation we evaluated beta-cell function relative to insulin sensitivity in black vs white children. Contrary to our expectation, our results revealed that the glucose DI is significantly higher in black children.[52] Even though insulin sensitivity is ~22% lower in blacks, glucose DI is ~75% higher. This suggests that for the same degree of insulin sensitivity, insulin secretion is higher in black children, as evident in Figure 6.2. The hyperinsulinemia observed in black children does not seem to be only a compensatory adaptation to lower insulin sensitivity. There seems to be an additional element of insulin hypersecretion.

We postulate that lifestyle dietary habits, particularly increased fat intake, through the effects of free fatty acids (FFAs) on insulin secretion, may play a role. In our study the higher fat/carbohydrate (CHO) ratio in the diet of black children correlated inversely with insulin sensitivity and clearance and positively with FFA levels and with first-phase insulin concentrations.[52] Black children have been reported to have high fat intake in some[53,54] but not all studies.[55] It remains to be determined if dietary habits are responsible for the lower insulin sensitivity and higher insulin secretion in black children. On the other hand, low levels of physical activity and fitness, which have been described in black children, may also play a role.[56–58] However, our observation (unpublished data) and those of others demonstrate that neither physical activity nor fitness could explain the black/white difference in insulin secretion and sensitivity.[58]

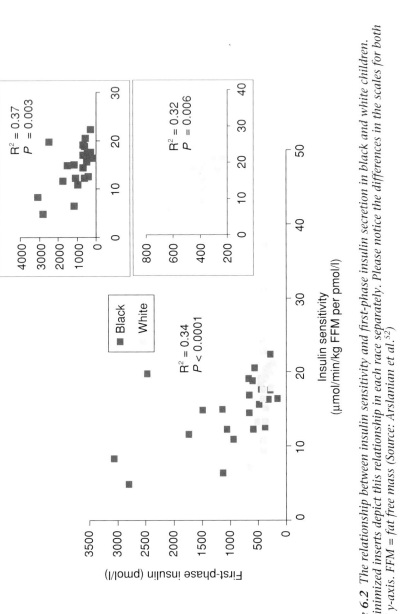

Figure 6.2 *The relationship between insulin sensitivity and first-phase insulin secretion in black and white children. The minimized inserts depict this relationship in each race separately. Please notice the differences in the scales for both x- and y-axis. FFM = fat free mass (Source: Arslanian et al.[52])*

Black/white differences in insulin sensitivity, secretion, and clearance have also been observed in adults.[59–61] In a nationally representative sample of adults (n = 6538) in the US population, blacks had higher fasting insulin levels, lower C-peptide values, and lower molar ratios of C-peptide/insulin compared with whites, suggestive of derangement in insulin clearance and impairment in beta-cell function.[61] Because alterations in insulin clearance, sensitivity, and secretion are detected early in the first decade of life in black children, interventions which modify the environmental impact on insulin sensitivity and secretion should be initiated early in childhood.

Puberty, insulin sensitivity, and secretion

The mean age of diagnosis of type 2 diabetes is 13.5 years, in mid puberty.[23–26,28,62–64] This could be related to the decrease in insulin action during puberty, which, in the case of a child with type 2 diabetes, further accentuates insulin resistance and the need for increased insulin secretion. The earliest information on the presence of insulin resistance during puberty came from studies evaluating changes in serum insulin concentrations related to hormonal changes of puberty. In 1975, Rosenbloom *et al.* demonstrated that insulin responses during an OGTT increase significantly from toddlerhood to adolescence in both healthy and glucose-intolerant individuals.[65] A year later, Lestradet *et al.* reported that in healthy children insulin levels during an OGTT were significantly elevated at the age of puberty compared with prepuberty.[66] Follow-up studies demonstrated that basal and stimulated insulin levels rose throughout puberty and declined following puberty until the third decade and remained constant thereafter.[67] Moreover, higher insulin concentrations were seen in those subjects who secreted the most growth hormone (GH), with a positive correlation between fasting insulin concentrations and height velocity.[68,69] Taken together, these results lead to the conclusion that there is a temporary physiological insulin resistance during puberty, manifested as hyperinsulinemia, driven by the elevations of GH during puberty, both of which subside after completion of puberty.

The direct evidence for pubertal insulin resistance became apparent only after using experiments which measure in-vivo insulin sensitivity. Amiel and colleagues, using the euglycemic insulin clamp, were the first to demonstrate that in nondiabetic and diabetic pubertal adolescents, insulin sensitivity was 25–30% lower compared with prepubertal children or adults.[70] Our studies show that the decrease in insulin-stimulated glucose disposal in adolescents involves both oxidative and nonoxidative glucose metabolism.[71] Competition between FFAs and glucose and increased lipid oxidation mediated by elevated GH may be responsible for pubertal insulin resistance.[71,72] The insulin resistance of puberty is limited to the peripheral tissues without affecting hepatic glucose production.[71–73] Similar observations of lower insulin sensitivity and higher insulinemia during puberty have been made by several other investigators using a variety of techniques, including the minimal model frequently sampled intravenous glucose tolerance test.[74–77] Consistent with the cross-sectional data, a longitudinal study of 31 children progressing from Tanner stage I puberty to Tanner stage III or IV showed that insulin sensitivity (tolbutamide-modified intravenous glucose tolerance test and minimal modeling) fell by ~30%.[78] In the presence of a normally functioning pancreatic beta cell, the puberty-related decrease in insulin sensitivity is compensated by increased insulin secretion demonstrated cross-sectionally and longitudinally.[78,79] However, when we investigated the impact of puberty in black children separately, despite ~30% lower insulin sensitivity in adolescents compared with prepubertal children, first- and second-phase insulin levels were not higher, unlike in white children (Figures 6.3 and 6.4).[80] This may suggest that in black children, despite prepubertal hyperinsulinemia, the pancreatic beta cell may have a limited capacity to further increase insulin secretion during puberty. Longitudinal studies, specifically in black children, are needed to further investigate this phenomenon. Whether or not this could explain the pubertal peak in onset of type 2 diabetes, particularly in black children, remains in question.

The cause of insulin resistance during puberty has been under investigation. Both GH and sex steroids are likely candidates; however, the transient nature of pubertal insulin resistance is out of tempo with the

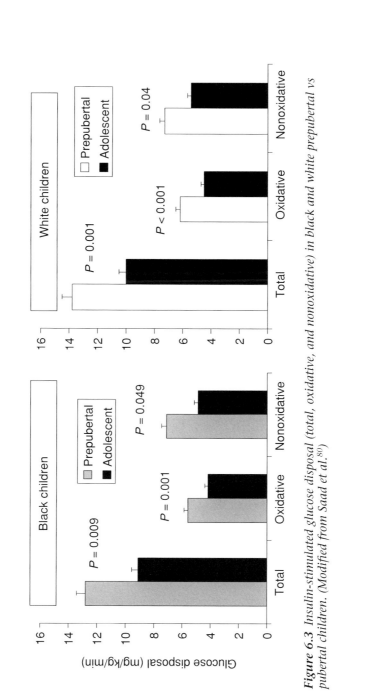

Figure 6.3 Insulin-stimulated glucose disposal (total, oxidative, and nonoxidative) in black and white prepubertal vs pubertal children. (Modified from Saad et al.[80])

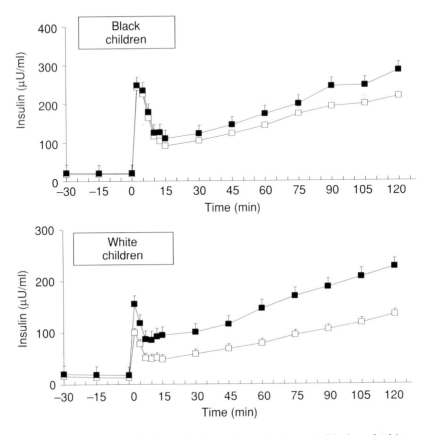

Figure 6.4 *Insulin levels during the hyperglycemic clamp in black and white prepubertal (open squares) vs pubertal (filled squares) children. (Modified from Saad et al.[80])*

increasing levels of sex steroids, which remain elevated in young adults while insulin resistance subsides. On the other hand, GH secretion increases during puberty coincident with the decrease in insulin action.[81] Studies have demonstrated that insulin-stimulated glucose metabolism correlates inversely with GH or insulin-like growth factor-I levels in white and black children.[70,71,80] Our research has shown that administering GH to adolescents with normal variant short stature who are not GH deficient, is associated with a deterioration in insulin action.[82] On the other hand, testosterone or dihydrotestosterone administration in boys with delayed puberty has no such effect.[83,84] Thus, increased GH secretion during normal puberty is most probably responsible for the insulin resistance that evolves during puberty, and both these changes subside with the completion of puberty.

Given this information, it is not surprising that the peak age at which youths present with type 2 diabetes is in mid-puberty at about 13.5 years. In an individual who has a genetic component of insulin resistance compounded by environmental factors, the additional burden of evolving insulin resistance during puberty may tip the balance from a state of compensated hyperinsulinemia with normal glucose tolerance to a decompensated state of beta-cell failure and glucose intolerance.

Family history of type 2 diabetes, insulin sensitivity, and secretion

A consistent finding in youth with type 2 diabetes is the presence of a first- or second-degree relative with type 2 diabetes. Among Pima Indians under the age of 25 years, diabetes occurs exclusively in persons with at least one diabetic parent.[13] Eighty percent of Hispanic youth have an affected first-degree relative and 47% have diabetes in three or more generations.[25] Among African-American youth with type 2 diabetes, 95% have a family history of type 2 diabetes, with multiple affected family members in more than one generation.[23,24]

Investigations of nondiabetic adult family members of patients with type 2 diabetes have shown abnormalities in both insulin action and beta-cell function. Insulin resistance precedes the development of type 2 diabetes by 1–2 decades in high-risk populations.[85,86] On the other hand, abnormalities in insulin secretion have also been described in subjects who are at high risk of developing type 2 diabetes. First-degree relatives of individuals with type 2 diabetes have diminished beta-cell function at a time when many of them still have normal glucose tolerance.[87,88] Our research in healthy black prepubertal children demonstrated that those children with a family history of type 2 diabetes have around 25% lower insulin sensitivity than those without such a family history despite comparable age, BMI, body composition, abdominal adiposity, and physical fitness levels.[89] This familial tendency for insulin resistance when combined with adverse environmental influences of high energy intake and low energy expenditure may result in type 2 diabetes years later. It remains to be determined if abnormalities in beta-cell function are also present in children at high risk for type 2 diabetes.

Polycystic ovary syndrome, insulin sensitivity, and secretion

Polycystic ovary syndrome, a common endocrinopathy affecting women in the reproductive age group, is being increasingly recognized in adolescent girls.[90] It is a heterogeneous disorder characterized by hyperandrogenism and oligo/amenorrhea secondary to chronic anovulation.[91] Associated clinical features include hirsutism, acne, and obesity. A major component of the syndrome is insulin resistance/hyperinsulinemia, which is present in both obese and lean adults with PCOS.[92] Adult women with PCOS are at increased risk for type 2 diabetes and impaired glucose tolerance (IGT).[93,94] Around 30% of adolescents with PCOS have IGT and ~4% have previously undiagnosed diabetes detected during OGTT.[95] Few studies in pediatrics have investigated insulin sensitivity and secretion in adolescents with PCOS. Limited reports show that adolescents with PCOS have fasting and stimulated hyperinsulinemia, and evidence of hepatic insulin resistance.[96,97]

In our studies insulin sensitivity was 50% lower in obese adolescents with PCOS compared with age, body composition, and abdominal obesity matched obese control girls.[98] In a follow-up study, we demonstrated that adolescents with PCOS who have IGT have 40% lower first-phase insulin secretion compared with those with normal glucose tolerance (NGT) (Figure 6.5).[99] In the presence of similar degrees of insulin resistance in the two groups, the lower first-phase insulin secretion resulted in a significantly lower glucose DI in the group with IGT (Figure 6.5).[99] These metabolic derangements are precursors of type 2 diabetes. Their presence early in the course of PCOS in the adolescent age group significantly increases their risk of type 2 diabetes if left without intervention. Metformin treatment for 3 months in obese adolescents with PCOS-IGT improved glucose tolerance and insulin sensitivity and lowered insulinemia and androgen

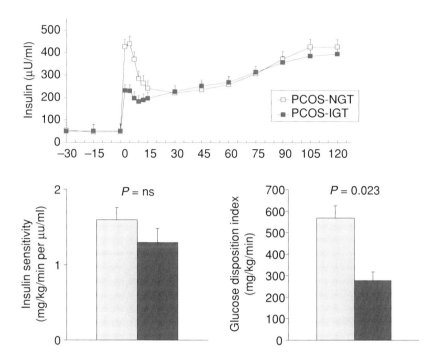

Figure 6.5 *Insulin secretion during a hyperglycemic clamp (upper panel), insulin sensitivity during a euglycemic clamp (left lower panel), and glucose disposition index (insulin sensitivity × first-phase insulin) (right lower panel) in polycystic ovary syndrome (PCOS) adolescents with normal glucose tolerance (PCOS-NGT) vs impaired glucose tolerance (PCOS-IGT). (Modified from Arslanian et al.[99])*

levels.[100] Large-scale double-blind placebo-controlled studies are needed to determine whether or not insulin-sensitizing therapy prevents and/or delays the conversion from IGT to type 2 diabetes in adolescents with PCOS.

Intrauterine growth retardation, insulin sensitivity, and secretion

Several studies have linked size at birth, or indices of poor fetal growth, with later development of impaired glucose tolerance and type 2 diabetes in adults.[101–103] This is postulated to be due to intrauterine 'programming', a term used to describe persistent changes in organ function caused by exposure to adverse in-utero environmental influences.[104]

Most of the studies showing that subjects with low birth weight are insulin resistant and predisposed to develop type 2 diabetes have been performed in adults.[105–108] Data in the pediatric literature are extremely limited, with most of the studies using indirect indexes of insulin action or secretion. In a study of 477 8-year-old Indian children, the association of lower birth weight with fasting insulin level reached statistical significance ($P = 0.08$).[109] Lower birth weight was associated with increased calculated HOMA (homeostasis model assessment) insulin resistance index but not HOMA beta-cell function.[109] In another small study of short prepubertal children with intrauterine growth retardation (IUGR), insulin sensitivity, measured with a modified frequently-sampled IVGTT, was significantly lower than in the control group with normal birth weight.[110] Moreover, HOMA insulin sensitivity was significantly related to overnight GH secretion in short children born small for gestational age.[111] None of these studies, however, used sensitive methods of assessing body composition and abdominal adiposity, which are important determinants of insulin sensitivity. In a study where body composition was assessed, low birth weight was significantly associated with increased visceral fat.[112] Moreover, a large-scale study of 10–11-year-old British school children demonstrated that obesity is a more powerful determinant of insulin level and insulin resistance than is size at birth.[113]

It is possible that fuel metabolism in a pregnant woman might exert a long-range effect on her offspring, predisposing to obesity and IGT. This is supported by the demonstration that excessive insulin secretion in utero is a predictor of both obesity and IGT in adolescent offspring of diabetic mothers.[114] Among Pima Indians, those with high birth weight were more obese at 5–29 years of age, and those with low birth weight were thinner but more insulin resistant relative to their body size than those of normal birth weight.[115] Data are not available in youth with type 2 diabetes with respect to the impact of birth weight on insulin sensitivity and secretion. The limited data in the pediatric literature open new opportunities for understanding the complex mix of genetic and environmental effects, prenatal and/or postnatal, underlying the diseases of under- and overnutrition and their relationship to insulin sensitivity/secretion. Much research is needed on the effect of the intrauterine environment on outcomes in childhood and adulthood.

Conclusions

Genetic and environmental factors modulate insulin sensitivity and secretion in children. The past few years have seen an emerging epidemic of type 2 diabetes in children. This rapid increase has occurred too quickly to be the result of an increased genetic pool. Environmental influences of calorically dense nutrition and a sedentary lifestyle appear to play a major role in the escalating rates of type 2 diabetes globally. Intervention and prevention modalities which would improve insulin action and maintain the balance between insulin sensitivity and secretion must be initiated early in childhood as part of normal growth and development. These strategies should target sociocultural, behavioral, nutritional, and lifestyle modifications to reduce not only the escalating rates of type 2 diabetes but also its complications.

Acknowledgment

This work was supported by United States Public Health Service grant RO1 HD27503, K24 HD01357, MO1-RR00084 General Clinical Research Center and Eli-Lilly and Company.

References

1. Kahn CR. Banting Lecture: insulin action, diabetogenes, and the cause of type II diabetes. *Diabetes* 1994; **43**:1066–84.
2. Elbein SC, Hoffman MD, Bragg KL, Mayorga RA. The genetics of NIDDM: an update. *Diabetes Care* 1994; **17**:1523–33.
3. Harris MI, Flegal KM, Cowie CC *et al*. Prevalence of diabetes, impaired fasting glucose, and impaired glucose tolerance in U.S. adults. The Third National Health and Nutrition Examination Survey, 1988–1994. *Diabetes Care* 1998; **21**:518–24.

4. Kahn SE, Prigeon RL, McCullough DK *et al*. Quantification of the relationship between insulin sensitivity and β-cell function in human subjects: evidence for a hyperbolic function. *Diabetes* 1993; **42**:1663–72.
5. Kahn SE. Regulation of β-cell function in vivo: from health to disease. *Diabetes Rev* 1996; **4**:372–89.
6. Kahn SE. The importance of β-cell failure in the development and progression of type 2 diabetes. *J Clin Endocrinol Metab* 2001; **86**:4047–58.
7. Elbein SC, Hasstedt SJ, Wegner K, Kahn SE. Heritability of pancreatic beta-cell function among nondiabetic members of Caucasian familial type 2 diabetic kindreds. *J Clin Endocrinol Metab* 1999; **84**:1398–403.
8. Ferrannini E. Insulin resistance is central to the burden of diabetes. *Diabetes/Metabolism Rev* 1997; **13**:81–6.
9. Taylor SI. Insulin resistance or insulin deficiency: which is the primary cause of NIDDM? *Diabetes* 1994; **43**:735–40.
10. Home PD. Insulin resistance is not central to the burden of diabetes. *Diabetes/Metabolism Rev* 1997; **13**:87–92.
11. Himsworth H. Diabetes mellitus: a differentiation into insulin-sensitive and insulin-insensitive types. *Lancet* 1936; **i**:127–30.
12. Reaven GM. Role of insulin resistance in the pathophysiology of non-insulin dependent diabetes mellitus. *Diabetes/Metabolism Rev* 1993; **9**:5–12S.
13. Knowler WC, Pettitt DJ, Saad MF, Bennett PH. Diabetes mellitus in the Pima Indians: incidence, risk factors and pathogenesis. *Diabetes Metab Rev* 1990; **6**:1–27.
14. Knowler WC, Saad MF, Pettitt DJ *et al*. Determinants of diabetes mellitus in the Pima Indians. *Diabetes Care* 1993; **16**:216–27.
15. Haffner SM, Stern MP, Mitchell BD *et al*. Incidence of Type II in Mexican Americans predicted by fasting insulin and glucose levels, obesity and body fat distribution. *Diabetes* 1990; **39**:283–8.
16. Lillioja S, Mott DM, Howard BV *et al*. Impaired glucose tolerance as a disorder of insulin action. Longitudinal and cross-sectional studies in Pima Indians. *N Engl J Med* 1988; **318**:1217–25.
17. Lillioja S, Nyomba BL, Saad MF *et al*. Exaggerated early insulin release and insulin resistance in a diabetes-prone population: a metabolic comparison of Pima Indians and Caucasians. *J Clin Endocrinol Metab* 1991; **73**:866–76.
18. Sicree RA, Zimmett PZ, King HOM, Coventry JS. Plasma-insulin response among Nauruans. Prediction of deterioration in glucose tolerance over 6 years. *Diabetes* 1987; **36**:179–86.
19. Porte Jr D. β-cells in type II diabetes mellitus. *Diabetes* 1991; **40**:166–80.
20. Polonsky KS, Sturis J, Bell GI. Non-insulin-dependent diabetes mellitus – a genetically programmed failure of the beta cell to compensate for insulin resistance. *N Engl J Med* 1996; **334**:777–83.
21. Porte D Jr. Clinical importance of insulin secretion and its interaction with insulin resistance in the treatment of type 2 diabetes mellitus and its complications. *Diabetes Metab Res Rev* 2001; **17**:181–8.
22. Arslanian S. Type 2 diabetes mellitus in children: pathophysiology and risk factors. *J Pediatr Endocrinol Metab* 2000; **13**:1385–94.
23. Pinhas-Hamiel O, Dolan LM, Daniels SR *et al*. Increased incidence of non-insulin-dependent diabetes mellitus among adolescents. *J Pediatr* 1996; **128**:608–15.

24. Scott CR, Smith JM, Cradock MM, Pihoker C. Characteristics of youth-onset non-insulin-dependent diabetes mellitus and insulin-dependent diabetes mellitus at diagnosis. *Pediatrics* 1997; **100**:84–91.
25. Glaser SN. Non-insulin-dependent diabetes mellitus in childhood and adolescence. *Pediatr Clin North Am* 1997; **44**:307–37.
26. Dean HJ. NIDDM-Y in First Nation children in Canada. *Clin Pediatr* 1998; **37**:89–96.
27. Rosenbloom AL, Joe JR, Young RS, Winter WE. Emerging epidemic of type 2 diabetes in youth. *Diabetes Care* 1999; **22**:345–54.
28. Dabelea D, Pettitt DJ, Jones KL, Arslanian SA. Type 2 diabetes mellitus in minority children and adolescents. An emerging problem. *Endocrinol Metab Clin N Am* 1999; **28**:709–29.
29. Ogden CL, Flegal KM, Carroll MD, Johnson CL. Prevalence and trends in overweight among US children and adolescents, 1999–2000. *JAMA* 2002; **288**:1728–32.
30. World Health Organization. Obesity: preventing and managing the global epidemic. Report of a WHO consultation. *World Health Organ Tech Rep Ser* 2000; **894**:i–xii,1–253.
31. Sorensen TI. The changing lifestyle in the world. Body weight and what else? *Diabetes Care* 2000; **23**:B1–4.
32. Pi-Sunyer FX. Health implications of obesity. *Am J Clin Nutr* 1991; **53**:15955–6035.
33. Caprio S, Tamborlane WV. Metabolic impact of obesity in childhood. *Endocrinol Metab Clin N Am* 1999; **28**:731–47.
34. DeCourten M, Bennett P, Tuomilehto J, Zimmet P. Epidemiology of NIDDM in non-Europids. In: Alberti KGMM, Zimmet PZ, DeFronzo RA, Keen H, eds. *International textbook of diabetes mellitus*, 2nd edn. London: John Wiley, 1997; 143–70.
35. Kissebah AH. Central obesity: measurement and metabolic effects. *Diab Rev* 1997; **5**:8–20.
36. Bonadonna RC, Bonora E. Glucose and free fatty acid metabolism in human obesity. Relationship to insulin resistance. *Diab Rev* 1997; **5**:21–51.
37. Arslanian S, Suprasongsin C. Insulin sensitivity, lipids and body composition in children: is 'syndrome X' present? *J Clin Endocrinol Metab* 1996; **81**:1058–62.
38. Goran MI, Bergman RN, Gower BA. Influence of total vs visceral fat on insulin action and secretion in African American and white children. *Obes Res* 2001; **9**:423–31.
39. Caprio S, Hyman LD, Limb C *et al.* Central adiposity and its metabolic correlates in obese adolescent girls. *Am J Physiol* 1995; **269**:E118–26.
40. Gower BA, Nagy TR, Goran MI. Visceral fat, insulin sensitivity and lipids in prepubertal children. *Diabetes* 1999; **48**:1515–21.
41. Caprio S, Bronson M, Sherwin RS *et al.* Co-existence of severe insulin resistance and hyperinsulinemia in preadolescent obese children. *Diabetologia* 1996; **39**:1489–97.
42. Kobayashi K, Amemiya S, Higashida K *et al.* Pathogenic factors of glucose intolerance in obese Japanese adolescents with type 2 diabetes. *Metabolism* 2000; **49**:186–91.

43. Legido A, Sarria A, Bueno M *et al.* Relationship of body fat distribution to metabolic complications in obese prepubertal boys: gender related differences. *Acta Paediatr Scand* 1989; **78**:440–6.
44. Umpaichitra V, Bastian W, Taha D *et al.* C-peptide and glucagons profiles in minority children with type 2 diabetes mellitus. *J Clin Endocrinol Metab* 2001; **86**:1605–9.
45. Svec F, Nastasi K, Hilton C, Bao W *et al.* Black–White contrasts in insulin levels during pubertal development. The Bogalusa Heart Study. *Diabetes* 1992; **41**:313–17.
46. Jiang X, Srinivasan SR, Radhakrishnamurthy B *et al.* Racial (Black–White) differences in insulin secretion and clearance in adolescents: The Bogalusa Heart Study. *Pediatrics* 1996; **97**:357–60.
47. Gutin B, Islam S, Manos T *et al.* Relation of percentage of body fat and maximal aerobic capacity to risk factors for atherosclerosis and diabetes in Black and White seven-to-eleven-year-old children. *J Pediatr* 1994; **125**:847–52.
48. Arslanian S, Suprasongsin C, Janosky JE. Insulin secretion and sensitivity in black versus white prepubertal healthy children. *J Clin Endocrinol Metab* 1997; **82**:1923–7.
49. Arslanian S, Suprasongsin C. Differences in the in vivo insulin secretion and sensitivity in healthy black vs white adolescents. *J Pediatr* 1996; **129**:440–4.
50. Gower BA, Nagy TR, Goran MI. Visceral fat, insulin sensitivity and lipids in prepubertal children. *Diabetes* 1999; **48**:1515–21.
51. Gower BA, Granger WM, Franklin F *et al.* Contribution of insulin secretion and clearance to glucose-induced insulin concentration in African-American and Caucasian children. *J Clin Endocrinol Metab* 2002; **87**:2218–24.
52. Arslanian SA, Saad R, Lewy V *et al.* Hyperinsulinemia in African-American children: decreased insulin clearance and increased insulin secretion and its relationship to insulin sensitivity. *Diabetes* 2002; **51**:3014–19.
53. Kimm SYS, Gergen PJ, Malloy M *et al.* Dietary patterns of US children: implications for disease prevention. *Prev Med* 1990; **19**:432–42.
54. Bacon AW, Miles JS, Schiffman SS. Effect of race on perception of fat alone and in combination with sugar. *Physiol Behav* 1994; **55**:603–6.
55. Lindquist CH, Gower BA, Goran MI. Role of dietary factors in ethnic differences in early risk of cardiovascular disease and type 2 diabetes. *Am J Clin Nutr* 2000; **71**:725–32.
56. Aaron DJ, Kriska AM, Dearwater SR *et al.* The epidemiology of leisure physical activity in an adolescent population. *Med Sci Sports Exerc* 1993; **25**:847–53.
57. Pivarnik JM, Bray MS, Hergenroeder AC *et al.* Ethnicity affects aerobic fitness in US adolescent girls. *Med Sci Sports Exerc* 1995; **27**:1635–8.
58. Ku CY, Gower BA, Hunter GR, Goran MI. Racial differences in insulin secretion and sensitivity in prepubertal children: role of physical fitness and physical activity. *Obes Res* 2000; **8**:506–15.
59. Osei K, Schuster DP, Owusu SK, Amoah AGB. Race and ethnicity determine serum insulin and C-peptide concentrations and hepatic insulin extraction and insulin clearance: comparative studies of three populations of West African ancestry and white Americans. *Metabolism* 1997; **46**:53–8.
60. Haffner SM, D'Agostino Jr R, Saad MF *et al.* Increased insulin resistance and insulin secretion in nondiabetic African-Americans and Hispanics compared

with non-Hispanic whites. The Insulin Resistance Atherosclerosis Study. *Diabetes* 1996; **45**:742–8.

61. Harris MI, Cowie CC, Gu K *et al*. Higher fasting insulin but lower fasting C-peptide levels in African Americans in the US population. *Diabetes Metab Res Rev* 2002; **18**:149–55.

62. Neufeld ND, Raffel LJ, Landon C *et al*. Early presentation of type 2 diabetes in Mexican-American youth. *Diabetes Care* 1998; **21**:80–6.

63. Ehtisham S, Barrett TG, Shaw NJ. Type 2 diabetes mellitus in UK children – an emerging problem. *Diab Med* 2000; **17**:867–71.

64. American Diabetes Association. Type 2 diabetes in children and adolescents. *Diabetes Care* 2000; **23**:381–9.

65. Rosenbloom AL, Wheeler L, Bianchi R *et al*. Age-adjusted analysis of insulin responses during normal and abnormal glucose tolerance tests in children and adolescents. *Diabetes* 1975; **24**:820–8.

66. Lestradet H, Deschamps I, Giron B. Insulin and free fatty acid levels during oral glucose tolerance tests and their relation to age in 70 healthy children. *Diabetes* 1976; **25**:505–8.

67. Smith CP, Williams AJK, Thomas JM *et al*. The pattern of basal and stimulated insulin responses to intravenous glucose in first degree relatives of Type 1 (insulin-dependent) diabetic children and unrelated adults aged 5 to 50 years. *Diabetologia* 1988; **31**:430–4.

68. Hindmarsh P, DiSilvio L, Pringle PJ *et al*. Changes in serum insulin concentration during puberty and their relationship to growth hormone. *Clin Endocrinol* 1988; **28**:381–8.

69. Hindmarsh PC, Matthews DR, DiSilvio L *et al*. Relation between height velocity and fasting insulin concentrations. *Arch Dis Childhood* 1988; **63**:665–6.

70. Amiel SA, Sherwin RS, Simenson DC *et al*. Impaired insulin action in puberty. *N Engl J Med* 1986; **315**:215–19.

71. Arslanian SA, Kalhan SC. Correlations between fatty acid and glucose metabolism: potential explanation of insulin resistance of puberty. *Diabetes* 1994; **43**:908–14.

72. Arslanian S, Suprasongsin C. Glucose–fatty acid interactions in prepubertal and pubertal children: effects of lipid infusion. *Am J Physiol* 1997; **272**: E523–9.

73. Amiel SA, Caprio S, Sherwin RS *et al*. Insulin resistance of puberty: a defect restricted to peripheral glucose metabolism. *J Clin Endocrinol Metab* 1991; **72**:277–82.

74. Block CA, Clemons P, Sperling MA. Puberty decreases insulin sensitivity. *J Pediatr* 1987; **110**:418–27.

75. Cook JS, Hoffman RP, Steine MA, Hansen JR. Effects of maturational stage on insulin sensitivity during puberty. *J Clin Endocrinol Metab* 1993; **77**:725–30.

76. Travers SH, Jeffers BW, Bloch CA *et al*. Gender and Tanner stage difference in body composition and insulin sensitivity in early pubertal children. *J Clin Endocrinol Metab* 1995; **80**:172–8.

77. Moran A, Jacobs DR Jr, Steinberger J *et al*. Insulin resistance during puberty. *Diabetes* 1999; **48**:2039–44.

78. Goran MI, Gower BA. Longitudinal study on pubertal insulin resistance. *Diabetes* 2001; **50**:2444–50.

79. Caprio S, Plewe G, Diamond MP *et al*. Increased insulin secretion in puberty: a compensatory response to reductions in insulin sensitivity. *J Pediatr* 1989; **114**:963–7.
80. Saad RJ, Danadian K, Lewy V, Arslanian SA. Insulin resistance of puberty in African-American children: lack of a compensatory increase in insulin secretion. *Pediatr Diab* 2002; **3**:4–9.
81. Metzger DL, Kerrigan JR, Rogol AD. Gonadal steroid hormone regulation of the somatotropic axis during puberty in humans: mechanisms of androgen and estrogen action. *Trends Endocrinol Metab* 1994; **5**:290–6.
82. Arslanian SA, Danadian K, Suprasongsin C. GH treatment in adolescents with non-GH deficient short stature (NGHD-SS): physical, biochemical and metabolic changes. *Pediatr Res* 1999; **45**(4):84A.
83. Arslanian S, Suprasongsin C. Testosterone treatment in adolescents with delayed puberty: changes in body composition, protein, fat, and glucose metabolism. *J Clin Endocrinol Metab* 1997; **82**:3213–20.
84. Saad RJ, Keenan BS, Danadian K *et al*. Dihydrotestosterone treatment in adolescents with delayed puberty: does it explain insulin resistance of puberty? *J Clin Endocrinol Metab* 2001; **86**:4881–6.
85. Warram JH, Martin BC, Krolewski AS *et al*. Slow glucose removal rate and hyperinsulinemia precede the development of type II diabetes in the offspring of diabetic parents. *Ann Intern Med* 1990; **113**:909–15.
86. Martin B, Warram JH, Krolewski AJ *et al*. Role of glucose and insulin resistance in development of type 2 diabetes mellitus: results of a 25-year follow-up study. *Lancet* 1992; **340**:925–9.
87. Ehrmann DA, Sturis J, Byrne MM *et al*. Insulin secretory defects in polycystic ovary syndrome. Relationship to insulin sensitivity and family history of non-insulin-dependent diabetes mellitus. *J Clin Invest* 1995; **96**:520–7.
88. Elbein SC, Wegner K, Kahn SE. Reduced β-cell compensation to the insulin resistance associated with obesity in members of Caucasian familial type 2 diabetic kindreds. *Diabetes Care* 2000; **23**:221–7.
89. Danadian K, Balasekaran G, Lewy V *et al*. Insulin sensitivity in African-American children with and without family history of Type 2 diabetes. *Diabetes Care* 1999; **22**:1325–9.
90. Arslanian SA, Witchel SF. Polycystic ovary syndrome in adolescents: is there an epidemic? *Curr Opin Endocrinol Diabetes* 2002; **9**:32–42.
91. Rosenfield RL. Ovarian and adrenal function in polycystic ovary syndrome. *Endocrinol Metab Clin N Am* 1999; **28**:265–93.
92. Dunaif A. Insulin resistance and the polycystic ovary syndrome: mechanism and implications for pathogenesis. *Endoc Rev* 1997; **18**:774–800.
93. Legro RS, Kunselman AR, Dodson WC *et al*. Prevalence and predictors of risk for type 2 diabetes mellitus and impaired glucose tolerance in polycystic ovary syndrome: a prospective, controlled study in 254 affected women. *J Clin Endocrinol Metab* 1999; **84**:165–9.
94. Ehrmann DA, Barnes RB, Rosenfield RL *et al*. Prevalence of impaired glucose tolerance and diabetes in women with polycystic ovary syndrome. *Diabetes Care* 1999; **22**:141–6.
95. Palmert MR, Gordon CM, Kartashov AI, Legro RS. Screening for abnormal glucose tolerance in adolescents with polycystic ovary syndrome. *J Clin Endocrinol Metab* 2002; **87**:1017–23.

96. Ibanez L, Potau N, Zampolli M *et al*. Hyperinsulinemia in postpubertal girls with a history of premature pubarche and functional ovarian hyperandrogenism. *J Clin Endocrinol Metab* 1996; **81**:1237–43.

97. Mauras N, Welch S, Rini A *et al*. Ovarian hyperandrogenism is associated with insulin resistance to both peripheral carbohydrate and whole-body protein metabolism in postpubertal young females: a metabolic study. *J Clin Endocrinol Metab* 1998; **83**:1900–5.

98. Lewy VD, Danadian K, Witchel SF *et al*. Early metabolic abnormalities in adolescent girls with polycystic ovarian syndrome. *J Pediatr* 2001; **138**:38–44.

99. Arslanian SA, Lewy VD, Danadian K. Glucose intolerance in obese adolescents with polycystic ovary syndrome: roles of insulin resistance and β-cell dysfunction and risk of cardiovascular disease. *J Clin Endocrinol Metab* 2001; **86**:66–71.

100. Arslanian SA, Lewy V, Danadian K, Saad R. Metformin therapy in obese adolescents with polycystic ovary syndrome and impaired glucose tolerance: amelioration of exaggerated adrenal response to adrenocorticotropin with reduction of insulinemia/insulin resistance. *J Clin Endocrinol Metab* 2002; **87**:1555–9.

101. Barker DJ, Hales CN, Fall CH *et al*. Type 2 (non-insulin-dependent) diabetes mellitus, hypertension and hyperlipidaemia (syndrome X): relation to reduced fetal growth. *Diabetologia* 1993; **36**:62–7.

102. Hales CN, Barker DJ. Type 2 (non-insulin-dependent) diabetes mellitus: the thrifty phenotype hypothesis. *Diabetologia* 1992; **35**:595–601.

103. Valdez R, Athens MA, Thompson GH *et al*. Birthweight and adult health outcomes in a biethnic population in the USA. *Diabetologia* 1994; **37**:624–31.

104. Lucas A. Role of nutritional programming in determining adult morbidity. *Arch Dis Childhood* 1994; **71**:288–90.

105. Hales CN, Barker DJ, Clark PM *et al*. Fetal and infant growth and impaired glucose tolerance at age 64. *BMJ* 1991; **303**:1019–22.

106. Lithell HO, McKeigue PM, Berglund L *et al*. Relation of size at birth to non-insulin dependent diabetes and insulin concentrations in men aged 50–60 years. *BMJ* 1996; **312**:406–10.

107. McKeigue PM, Lithell HO, Leon DA. Glucose tolerance and resistance to insulin-stimulated glucose uptake in men aged 70 years in relation to size at birth. *Diabetologia* 1998; **41**:1133–8.

108. Rosenbloom AL. Fetal and childhood nutrition in type 2 diabetes in children and adults. *Pediatr Diab* 2000; **1**:34–40.

109. Bavdekar A, Yajnik CS, Fall CHD *et al*. Insulin resistance syndrome in 8-year-old Indian children: small at birth, big at 8 years, or both? *Diabetes* 1999; **48**:2422–9.

110. Hofman PL, Cutfield WS, Robinson EM *et al*. Insulin resistance in short children with intrauterine growth retardation. *J Clin Endocrinol Metab* 1997; **82**:402–6.

111. Woods KA, VanHelvoirt M, Ong KKL *et al*. The somatotropic axis in short children born small for gestational age: relation to insulin resistance. *Pediatr Res* 2002; **51**:76–80.

112. Li C, Johnson MS, Goran MI. Effects of low birth weight on insulin resistance syndrome in Caucasian and African-American children. *Diabetes Care* 2001; **24**(12):2035–42.

113. Whincup PH, Cook DG, Adshead F *et al*. Childhood size is more strongly related than size at birth to glucose and insulin levels in 10–11 year old children. *Diabetologia* 1997; **40**:319–26.
114. Silverman BL, Rizzo TA, Cho NH, Metzger BE. Long-term effects of the intrauterine environment. *Diabetes Care* 1998; **21**:142–9.
115. Dabelea D, Pettitt DJ, Hanson RL *et al*. Birthweight, type 2 diabetes, and insulin resistance in Pima Indian children and young adults. *Diabetes Care* 1999; **22**:944–50.

chapter 7

In-utero undernutrition and glucose homeostasis later in life

Delphine Jaquet, Claire Lévy-Marchal, and Paul Czernichow

Introduction

Evidence over the past 10 years has demonstrated a significant association between reduced fetal growth and the later development of metabolic and cardiovascular diseases.

Knowledge from epidemiological studies

The unexpected long-term deleterious effect of reduced fetal growth was initially observed by Barker and colleagues. This group first reported that a low birth weight was significantly associated with an increased risk for the later development of cardiovascular diseases or type 2 diabetes in a cohort of Caucasian males aged 64 years.[1,2] Other epidemiological studies performed in Pima Indians or in Caucasian subjects later confirmed this observation, suggesting that the association holds true whether the study populations are genetically predisposed or not to type 2 diabetes.[3,4]

The independent effect of thinness at birth, assessed by the ponderal index, and the lack of association with gestational age on these complications observed in several studies support the hypothesis of deleterious effect of reduced fetal growth rather than prematurity on this association.[2,4]

Numerous epidemiological studies have demonstrated that being born with a low birth weight is also associated with hypertension[1,5] or dyslipidemia.[6,7] These complications are clustered in syndrome X, which is initially described by Reaven as constituting a major cardiovascular risk factor.[8] Interestingly, Barker and colleagues reported that a low birth weight was also associated with a risk for the development of syndrome X in adulthood.[7] At 50 years of age the risk for the development of syndrome X was 10-fold higher in subjects with a birth weight less than 2.5 kg compared with subjects weighing 4.5 kg or more.[7] This association was independent of the current body weight or the gestational age. This observation was later confirmed in a US study population composed of Hispanic and non-Hispanic white subjects aged 30 years or more.[9] In this study population, the relative risk for the development of syndrome X increased 1.72 times for each tertile decrease in birth weight.

Mechanisms underlying this association

The Barker group initially proposed that type 2 diabetes could be the consequence of undernutrition occurring during a critical period of fetal life, with a consequent abnormal development of endocrine pancreas leading to an impaired beta-cell function.[2] They later extended this hypothesis to all the other organs involved in the development of the cardiovascular and metabolic abnormalities observed in syndrome X (also known as 'the metabolic syndrome'). Further epidemiological studies have failed to confirm this hypothesis and the mechanisms underlying the development of the metabolic complications associated with reduced fetal growth remain to be understood. However, the alternative approaches and the physiological investigations undertaken during the past few years have helped to clarify the pathophysiology of this clinical association.

In the early studies, birth data were retrospectively analyzed according to the metabolic profile observed in adulthood, and reduced fetal growth assessed by birth weight irrespective of gestational age, which was not available, introducing a confounding factor with prematurity. To specifically address the question of the metabolic consequences of fetal growth retardation and understand the possible mechanisms, an alternative approach has been to compare aged-matched subjects selected on birth data in a case/control study design in which subjects were born either small or appropriate for gestational age. Additionally, studies performed in subjects of different ages have allowed a better understanding of the chronological organization of the different components of the metabolic complications which might be associated with reduced fetal growth.

Which is the primary defect responsible for type 2 diabetes associated with reduced fetal growth?

Role of insulin resistance

The hypothesis of a critical role of insulin resistance in the metabolic complications associated with in-utero undernutrition has been well documented during the past few years. This hypothesis was firstly proposed by the San Antonio, Texas group, which pointed out the importance of insulin resistance in this association.[9] Insulin resistance has been proposed to be the central pathological process underlying the development of syndrome X.[10] It was therefore tempting to speculate that the clustering of these complications associated with reduced fetal growth involves primarily the development of insulin resistance.

The significant association between a low birth weight and hyperinsulinemia in adulthood observed in several epidemiological studies strongly suggests the development of insulin resistance.[2,4,7] Moreover, studies using the euglycemic hyperinsulinemic clamp method have demonstrated that type 2 diabetes associated with a low birth weight requires insulin resistance as described in the classical form of type 2 diabetes.[11]

In a case/control study, young adults (20 years old) born small for gestational age (SGA) demonstrated hyperinsulinemia in an oral glucose tolerance test (OGTT) compared with age-matched subjects born with normal birth size[12] (Figure 7.1). Reduced insulin sensitivity was present as early as 20 years of age in subjects born SGA using the euglycemic hyperinsulinemic clamp method[13] (Figure 7.2). Subjects born SGA demonstrated a peripheral glucose uptake significantly decreased in comparison to controls. Similar results were obtained using the minimal model.[14] These observations indicate the early development of insulin resistance in this situation.

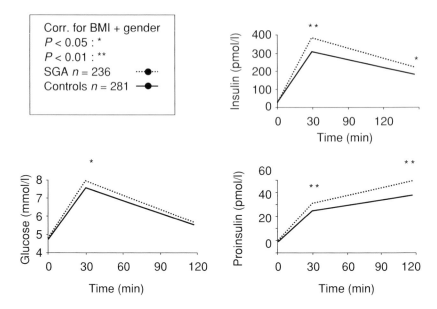

Figure 7.1 *Serum insulin, proinsulin, and plasma glucose concentrations during an OGTT (oral glucose tolerance test) in 20-year-old subjects who had been born SGA (small for gestational age) and control subjects.[12] Subjects born SGA demonstrated significantly higher insulin and proinsulin excursions during an OGTT than age-matched controls, suggesting the development of insulin resistance early in adulthood. BMI = body mass index.*

Both glucose oxidation and non-oxidative disposal rates were affected in the insulin resistance associated with reduced fetal growth.[15] These meta-bolic abnormalities are consistent with the impaired regulation by insulin of GLUT4 mRNA expression observed in muscle and adipose tissue of insulin-resistant subjects born SGA.[15] However, a similar impairment of GLUT4 expression has also been reported in other clinical situations associated with insulin resistance. This suggests that insulin resistance itself, rather than reduced fetal growth, is responsible for this abnormality. On the other hand, when subjects born SGA were compared to controls, there was no difference in the expression of the genes of the principal molecules described in the insulin-signaling pathway.[15] These observations were made under basal condition and after insulin stimulation both in muscle and adipose tissue.

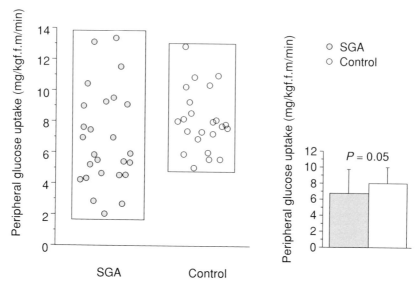

Figure 7.2 *Individual (left graph) and mean values (right graph) of peripheral glucose uptake under euglycemic hyperinsulinemic clamp in 24-year-old SGA (small for gestational age) adults (n = 25) and controls (n = 26) subjects.[13] Insulin resistance in subjects born SGA was confirmed by the significantly lower mean value of peripheral glucose uptake under euglycemic hyperinsulinemic (40 U/m²/min) clamp in comparison to controls. However, subjects born SGA showed scattered individual values of peripheral glucose uptake, suggesting a variable predisposition to insulin resistance. (f.f.m = fat-free mass)*

Hyperinsulinemia was the only feature of the syndrome X present in subjects born SGA at the age of 20 years,[12,13] suggesting that, as in the syndrome X, insulin resistance could be the early critical component of the metabolic syndrome associated with reduced fetal growth. However, it should be emphasized that, clearly insulin-resistant SGA subjects already demonstrated minor lipid profile abnormalities or increased adiposity.[13]

Reduced fetal growth and beta-cell function (Table 7.1)

Insulin-secretion defect is the other major component of type 2 diabetes. It has been initially proposed that type 2 diabetes associated with a low birth weight could be the consequence of impaired beta-cell function as a result of undernutrition during a critical period of fetal life, leading to the abnormal development of the endocrine

Table 7.1 Evidence against or in favor of a beta-cell dysfunction associated with reduced fetal growth

Observations	Con	Pro
Humans		
Biological parameters:		
Robinson et al.[16]		Insulin secretion defect at 21 years of age (OGTT)
Léger et al.[12]	No insulin-secretion defect at 20 years of age (OGTT)	
Flanagan et al.[14]	Reduced insulin sensitivity compensated by increased insulin secretion at 20 years of age (minimal model)	
Jaquet et al.[13]	First-phase insulin release adapted to insulin sensitivity at 24 years of age (IVGTT)	
Jensen et al.[19]		Early differential defect of insulin secretion at 19 years of age (minimal model)
Jaquet et al.[20]	Normal insulin response during the first and the second phase under hyperglycemic clamp	
Anatomopathological parameters:		
Van Assche et al.[17]		Abnormal endocrine pancreas development in SGA fetuses
Béringue et al.[18]	Normal pancreas development and morphology in SGA fetuses in comparison to fetuses appropriate for gestational age	

Table 7.1 *Continued*

Observations	Con	Pro
Animal models		
Garofano et al.[24]		Impairment of beta-cell development in malnourished rats
Garofano et al.[25]		Impairment of beta-cell mass and function with aging in rats malnourished during the perinatal period

SGA = small for gestational age, OGTT = oral glucose tolerance test, IVGTT = intravenous glucose tolerance test.

pancreas.[2] Indeed, the same group later reported OGTT analyses showing that a low birth weight was associated with insulin-secretion defect in 21-year-olds.[16] Twenty-five years ago, an anatopathological study had reported an abnormal pancreas development in fetuses with severe intrauterine growth retardation.[17] However, it has recently been shown that SGA does not alter fetal pancreas development and morphology in comparison to fetuses with appropriate growth for gestational age (AGA) (Figure 7.3).[18] In a case/control study comparing

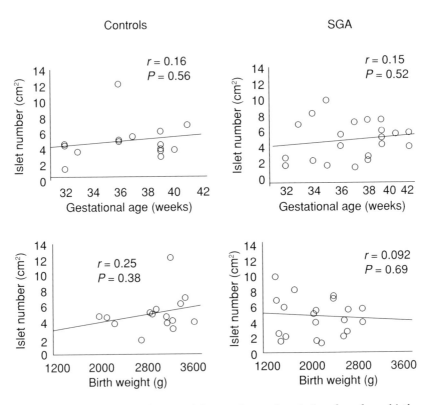

Figure 7.3 *Relationship between islet number and gestational weeks or birth weight in fetuses born small (SGA) or appropriate for gestational age (controls).[18] No significant relationship was observed between islet density and either gestational age or birth weight in SGA and control fetuses. Islet density does not appear to be altered by reduced fetal growth.*

young adults who had been born SGA or AGA, subjects born SGA did not show any evidence in favor of an insulin-secretion defect either under OGTT or using the minimal model.[12,14] In these subjects, the acute insulin response to an intravenous glucose tolerance test was adapted to the degree of insulin sensitivity, suggesting preservation of beta-cell function at the age of 20–25 years[13,14] (Figure 7.4). However, another group using a comparable study design recently reported that 19-year-old subjects born SGA showed differential defect of insulin secretion with respect to insulin action.[19] When measured under hyperglycemic clamp, young adults born SGA did not demonstrate impairment of insulin secretion, either during the first or the second

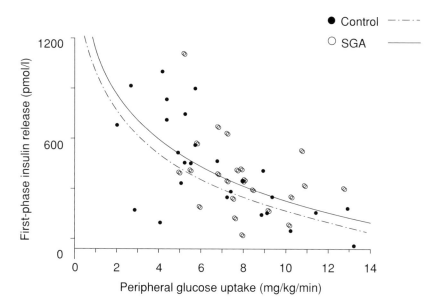

Figure 7.4 Relationship between the peripheral glucose uptake under euglycemic hyperinsulinemic clamp and the first-phase insulin release under IVGTT (intravenous glucose tolerance test) in 24-year-old SGA (small for gestational age) (n = 25) and control (n = 26) subjects.[13] The relationship between the peripheral glucose uptake and the first-phase insulin release under IVGTT was similar in both groups. This similarity strongly suggests that insulin response in young adults born SGA was adapted to the degree of insulin resistance.

phase.[20] Thus, impaired beta-cell function observed in type 2 diabetes associated with reduced fetal growth appears as a consequence of insulin resistance rather than a primary defect. Insulin resistance may contribute to beta-cell dysfunction in the common form of type 2 diabetes by gluco- or lipotoxicity.[21,22] Moreover, it has recently been shown that the tissue-specific knock-out of the insulin receptor in the beta cells leads to a beta-cell defect, suggesting that the insulin-secretion defect could reflect insulin resistance of the beta cells.[23] However, we cannot exclude some undetectable and minor beta-cell dysfunction, however, which in turn would be amplified by insulin resistance. In animal models, perinatal undernutrition is associated with an abnormal pancreas development and beta-cell function in adulthood.[24,25]

Are glucose homeostasis abnormalities already present in childhood?

Insulin resistance in childhood

Several epidemiological studies performed in children and adolescents suggest that minor glucose homeostasis abnormalities can be detected in childhood. Indian children with a birth weight less than 2.4 kg tend to have higher plasma glucose and serum insulin concentrations than children born heavier, as early as 4 years of age.[26] Studies performed in children from different ethnic groups (Pima Indians, Caucasians, Indians) showed that reduced fetal growth is associated with hyperinsu-linemia at fast or during OGTT and with decreased insulin sensitivity when measured with the minimal model.[27–29]

As in adults, the decreased insulin sensitivity associated with reduced fetal growth is not associated with evidence for a beta-cell defect in pre-pubertal children.[28] This observation strengthens the hypothesis that insulin resistance is the earliest critical component of the metabolic abnormalities associated with reduced fetal growth.

Respective contribution of birth size and current body sizes

Although reduced fetal growth has been shown to be an independent risk factor for the later development of metabolic complications, insulin resistance is sharply potentiated by obesity in children as in adults (Figure 7.5).[30] A study performed in 10–11-year-old children demonstrated that the proportional change in insulin level at fast and after glucose load for one SD increase in childhood ponderal index was much greater than that for birth weight (27.8% vs −8.8%, respectively, at fasting).[31] In a cohort of African American adolescents, peripheral glucose uptake did not significantly correlate with birth weight when current body weight was taken into account.[32] These data point to the crucial role of current body size in the risk for the

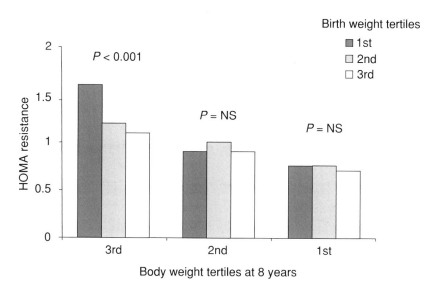

Figure 7.5 *Mean level of insulin resistance variable (HOMA) (adjusted for age and gender) at 8 years of age by tertiles of birth weight and current body weight.[28] This figure illustrates the interaction between size at birth and current body size on insulin-resistance parameters in childhood. As shown on the left of the figure, the more insulin-resistant subjects were the lightest at birth and the heaviest at 8 years of age.*

development of the metabolic abnormalities associated with reduced fetal growth. They also raise the question of the contribution of adiposity in this clinical association.

What role could adipose tissue play in this situation?

If insulin resistance is the primary defect responsible for metabolic abnormalities following reduced fetal growth, the mechanism should be sought among those factors directly responsible for the development of insulin resistance. An important contribution of adipose tissue seems to be a reasonable hypothesis.

Adipose tissue plays a key role in the development and the worsening of insulin resistance and its complications. The strong interaction between these two components is well demonstrated by the close relationship existing between obesity and the development of syndrome X.

Reduced fetal growth and adipose tissue development

Reduced fetal growth severely alters the perinatal development of adipose tissue. SGA newborns have a dramatically reduced body fat mass at birth.[33,34] This reduction mostly reflects a decreased fat accumulation in the adipocytes, as suggested by the low triglyceride content.[35] Most of these newborns, however, will show a catch-up growth during infancy.[36] This catch-up growth also involves the adipose tissue, as demonstrated by the sharp increase in body mass index (BMI) during the first year of life.[37] There is now accumulating evidence that the increased growth velocity of the adipose tissue could persist beyond catch-up. Ravelli *et al.*[38] first reported, over 25 years ago, that in-utero undernutrition could favor obesity in adulthood. More recently, it has been shown that children born SGA who had catch-up growth during infancy showed an increased body fat mass with a more central fat distribution in comparison to children born AGA.[39] Interestingly, another study has shown that despite being smaller than

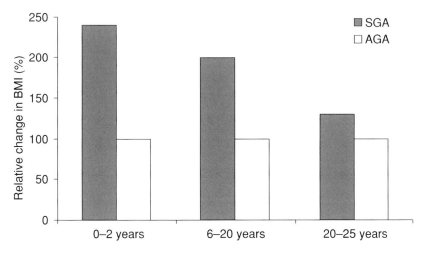

Figure 7.6 *Relative change in BMI (body mass index) from birth to early adulthood in subjects born SGA (small for gestational age) in comparison to age-matched subjects born AGA (appropriate growth for gestational age).[37,41,42] This figure illustrates the catch-up growth of adiposity from birth to adulthood in subjects born SGA in comparison to the physiological increase of BMI observed in subjects born AGA. For each period, change in BMI in the SGA group is expressed relatively to what is observed in the AGA group (with an assigned value at 100%).*

children born AGA, young children born SGA have a relatively increased percentage of body fat mass than children with normal birth size[40] (Figure 7.6). This would suggest that reduced fetal growth and the subsequent catch-up would alter body composition. The persistent catch-up of adiposity until adulthood is suggested by the relative increase of BMI throughout childhood observed in subjects born SGA and their significantly increased percentage of body fat mass at age 25 years in comparison to controls[37,41,42] (Figure 7.6).

Reduced fetal growth and adipose tissue hormonal functions

The abnormal development of adiposity in children born SGA is associated with hormonal and metabolic abnormalities. Insulin resistance observed in young adults born SGA also involves the adipose tissue.[13] In these subjects

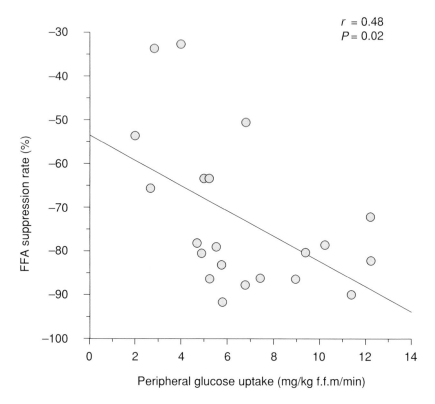

Figure 7.7 Relationship between peripheral glucose uptake and suppression rate of FFA (free fatty acids) under euglycemic hyperinsulinemic clamps in subjects born SGA (small for gestational age).[13] The close relationship existing in subjects born SGA between peripheral glucose uptake and FFA suppression rate under euglycemic hyperinsulinemic clamp illustrates the decreased antilipolytic action of insulin associated with insulin resistance. No such correlation was observed in age-matched controls. This observation argues in favor of the involvement of adipose tissue in the insulin resistance associated with reduced fetal growth. (f.f.m = fat-free mass)

the peripheral glucose uptake under the euglycemic hyperinsulinemic clamp closely correlates with the antilipolytic action of insulin assessed by changes in free fatty acid production during the clamp[13] (Figure 7.7).

Serum leptin concentrations are significantly reduced in SGA newborns and this reduction closely correlates with the reduced body fat mass.[34] However, leptin production and regulation appear to be altered by the catch-up growth of adipose tissue, with significantly higher serum leptin concentrations with respect to BMI in young children born SGA.[37] In contrast, adults born SGA showed lower serum leptin concentrations in comparison to controls with adjustment for gender, body fat mass, and serum insulin concentrations.[42] Although the mechanism of this dysregulation remains to be clarified, these observations are of interest because leptin, a regulator of body fat mass, is involved in the control of insulin sensitivity.

Taken together, these data argue in favor of an active contribution of adipose tissue in the insulin resistance associated with reduced fetal growth:

1. because the abnormal development of adipose tissue is, in this situation, leading to an increased body fat mass in adulthood, and could favor the development of such a syndrome, and
2. because this adipose tissue has dysregulated metabolic functions that could alter insulin sensitivity.

What is the origin of the development of insulin resistance associated with reduced fetal growth (Figure 7.8)?

Although the involvement of adipose tissue in the insulin resistance associated with reduced fetal growth is strongly suggested by the above observations, the origin of this association remains unclear. Two major hypotheses emerged from the initial epidemiological studies, both arising from the original theory of the 'thrifty genotype' proposed by Neel in 1962.[43] To explain the high prevalence of type 2 diabetes in Western populations, Neel hypothesized that genes that would favor survival during periods of famine would become detrimental when food supply became abundant and continuous. This theory encompasses the two major components of the association: undernutrition and the later development of metabolic complications.

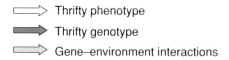

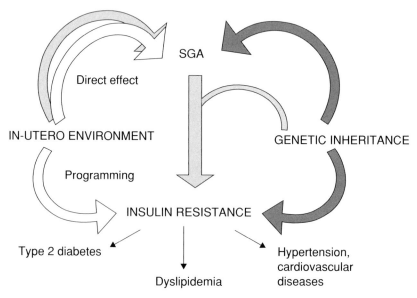

Figure 7.8 *Hypotheses proposed to explain the origin of the development of insulin resistance associated with reduced fetal growth. SGA = small for gestational age.*

'Thrifty phenotype hypothesis'

Hales *et al.*[2] proposed an alternative to the 'thrifty genotype' hypothesis – the 'thrifty phenotype' hypothesis – in which environmental factors play a critical role. According to the 'programming' process,[44] they proposed that 'alteration in fetal nutrition and endocrine status resulted in developmental adaptations that permanently change structure, physiology and metabolism, thereby predisposing individuals to cardiovascular, metabolic and endocrine diseases in adult life'.

'Thrifty genotype hypothesis'

From data collected in Pima Indians, McCance et al.[3] proposed another alternative to the 'thrifty genotype' and the 'thrifty phenotype': 'the surviving small baby genotype'. They hypothesized that given the high mortality associated with reduced fetal growth, selective survival of children genetically predisposed to insulin resistance and type 2 diabetes provides an explanation for this association. This hypothesis favors the genetic contribution. More recently, the same group reported data to support this hypothesis: in Pima Indians, a strong relationship was observed between a low birth weight in children and an increased prevalence of type 2 diabetes in their fathers, suggesting a paternal inheritance of genes controlling either fetal growth or glucose homeostasis.[45] In keeping with the idea of a genetic contribution, Hattersley and Tooke[46] proposed the 'fetal insulin hypothesis', suggesting that a genetically determined insulin resistance could result in a low insulin-mediated fetal growth as well as insulin resistance in childhood and adulthood. Indeed, it has been shown that several genetic polymorphisms, such as insulin gene VNTR and insulin-like growth factor-1 (IGF-1)-promoter polymorphism, could be associated with either type 2 diabetes or decreased birth weight.[47,48]

'Genotype–phenotype interaction'

However, these metabolic complications are known to result from both genetic and environmental factors in humans. Since neither the thrifty genotype hypothesis nor the thrifty phenotype hypothesis has been confirmed, it is tempting to speculate that both genetic and environmental factors together influence the development of the metabolic syndrome associated with reduced fetal growth. Thus, this association could be the consequence of interactions between detrimental environmental factors during fetal life and a genetic susceptibility, as initially proposed by the San Antonio group.[9] Epidemiological studies performed on mono- and dizygotic twins have demonstrated the effect of environmental and genetic factors on the development of the metabolic complications associated with reduced fetal growth.[49,50]

Is insulin resistance the only hormonal dysfunction responsible for the metabolic complications associated with reduced fetal growth?

Hypothalamo–pituitary–adrenal axis

Cortisol has been shown to decrease insulin sensitivity.[51] Additionally, insulin resistance and obesity are associated with a pituitary–adrenal axis hyperactivity.[52,53] On the other hand, steroid metabolism, involving the mother, the placenta, and the fetus, plays a critical role in fetal growth and development. It has been speculated that the hypothalamo–pituitary– adrenal axis might be involved in the glucose metabolism abnormalities associated with reduced fetal growth. Indeed, Phillips et al.[54] have shown that low birth weight is associated with elevated fasting cortisol in three different cohorts of Caucasian subjects aged 20–70 years. In these subjects fasting cortisol concentration was highly correlated with blood pressure although this correlation was more evident in obese subjects. It has been proposed that the glucose home-ostasis abnormalities associated with reduced fetal growth might result from the impairment of the pituitary–adrenal axis.[54,55] However, this hypothesis has not been validated. Additionally, results appear less con-vincing in pediatric ages. Clark et al.[56] have shown a weak U-shaped rela-tionship between birth weight and steroid urinary metabolites in prepubertal children. Using a case/control approach Dahlgren et al.[57] did not report significant differences in fasting cortisol concentration, corti-sol area under the curve, circadian rhythm, and response to adrenocorti-cotropic hormone (ACTH) between prepubertal short SGA ($n = 53$), short AGA ($n = 75$), and normal-sized AGA ($n = 56$) children. Further investiga-tion is needed of the interplay between serum cortisol concentration, adiposity, and insulin resistance.

Precocious pubarche, hyperandrogenism, and insulin resistance associated with reduced fetal growth

Precocious pubarche has been shown by Ibañez et al.[58,59] to be associ-ated with an increased frequency of postpubertal functional ovarian hyperandrogenism and hyperinsulinemia. They also reported that post-pubertal girls who exhibited the complete triad (precocious puberty, hyperandrogenism, and hyperinsulinemia) had birth weights significantly lower than postpubertal controls.[60] Consequently, it was hypothesized that this triad may result from a common early origin in reduced fetal growth.[60] In a study performed on 130 young women born with intrauterine growth retardation (IUGR) and 150 controls, women born with IUGR did not show any clinical or biological evidence of hyperandrogenism despite the presence of hyperinsulinemia.[61] The different selection criteria used in the two studies might explain the discrepancies. It cannot be excluded that the triad reported by Ibañez *et al.* might be associated in these girls with a decrease in birth weight due to a mechanism that remains to be clarified. However, from a broader point of view, being born with IUGR does not appear to favor hyperandrogenism in adulthood. This conclusion is consistent with the lack of relationship between a low birth weight and the later development of polycystic ovarian syndrome observed in a cohort of 42-year-old women.[62]

Conclusion

Investigations performed during the past 15 years have identified the independent association between reduced fetal growth and the later development of metabolic and cardiovascular complications. Using a prospective research program based on case control studies, our group has shown that the early development of insulin resistance in adulthood seems to be the key component underlying this unexpected association. Although the mechanism responsible for the development of insulin resistance in this situation remains unclear, we collected some evidence in favor of an active contribution by adipose tissue. From a broader point of view, the hypothesis suggesting that this association could be the consequence of interactions between a detrimental fetal environment and a genetic susceptibility remains most attractive but needs to be confirmed.

References

1. Barker DJ, Osmond C, Golding J *et al*. Growth in utero, blood pressure in childhood and adult life, and mortality from cardiovascular disease. *Br Med J* 1989; **298**:564–7.
2. Hales CN, Barker DJ, Clark PM *et al*. Fetal and infant growth and impaired glucose tolerance at age 64. *Br Med J* 1991; **303**:1019–22.
3. McCance DR, Pettitt DJ, Hanson RL *et al*. Birth weight and non-insulin dependent diabetes: thrifty genotype, thrifty phenotype, or surviving small baby genotype? *Br Med J* 1994; **308**:942–5.
4. Lithell HO, McKeigue PM, Berglund L *et al*. Relation of size at birth to non-insulin dependent diabetes and insulin concentrations in men aged 50–60 years. *Br Med J* 1996; **312**:406–10.
5. Leon DA, Koupilova I, Lithell HO *et al*. Failure to realize growth potential in utero and adult obesity in relation to blood pressure in 50 year old Swedish men. *Br Med J* 1996; **312**:401–6.
6. Barker DJP, Martyn CN, Osmond C *et al*. Growth in utero and serum cholesterol concentrations in adult life. *Br Med J* 1993; **207**:1524–7.
7. Barker DJ, Hales CN, Fall CH *et al*. Type 2 (non-insulin-dependent) diabetes mellitus, hypertension and hyperlipidaemia (syndrome X): relation to reduced fetal growth. *Diabetologia* 1993; **36**:62–7.
8. Reaven G. Role of insulin-resistance in human disease. *Diabetes* 1988; **37**:1595–607.
9. Valdez R, Athens MA, Thompson GH *et al*. Birthweight and adult health outcomes in a biethnic population in the USA. *Diabetologia* 1994; **37**:624–31.
10. Haffner SM, Valdez RA, Hazuda HP *et al*. Prospective analysis of the insulin-resistance syndrome (syndrome X). *Diabetes* 1992; **41**:715–22.
11. McKeigue PM, Lithell HO, Leon DA. Glucose tolerance and resistance to insulin-stimulated glucose uptake in men aged 70 years in relation to size at birth. *Diabetologia* 1998; **41**:1133–8.
12. Léger J, Lévy-Marchal C, Bloch J *et al*. Reduced final height and indications for insulin resistance in 20 year olds born small for gestational age: regional cohort study. *Br Med J* 1997; **315**:341–7.
13. Jaquet D, Gaboriau A, Czernichow P, Lévy-Marchal C. Insulin resistance early in adulthood in subjects born with intra-uterine growth retardation. *J Clin Endocrinol Metab* 2000; **85**:1401–6.
14. Flanagan DE, Moore VM, Godsland IF *et al*. Fetal growth and the physiological control of glucose tolerance in adults: a minimal model analysis. *Am J Physiol Endocrinol Metab* 2000; **208**:E700–6.
15. Jaquet D, Vidal H, Hankard R *et al*. Impaired regulation of GLUT-4 gene expression in insulin-resistance associated with in-utero undernutrition. *J Clin Endocrinol Metab* 2001; **86**:3266–71.
16. Robinson S, Walton RJ, Clark PM *et al*. The relation of fetal growth to plasma glucose in young men. *Diabetologia* 1992; **35**:444–6.
17. Van Assche FA, De Prins F, Aerts L, Verjans M. The endocrine pancreas in small-for-dates infants. *Br J Obstet Gynaecol* 1977; **84**:751–3.
18. Béringue F, Blondeau B, Castellotti MC *et al*. Endocrine pancreas development in growth retarded human foetuses. *Diabetes* 2002; **51**:385–91.

19. Jensen CB, Storgaart H, Dela F *et al*. Early differential defects of insulin-secretion and action in 19-year-old Caucasian men who had low birth weight. *Diabetes* 2002; **51**:1271–80.
20. Jaquet D, Chevenne D, Czernichow P, Lévy-Marchal C. No evidence for a major β-cell dysfunction in young adults born with intra-uterine growth retardation. *Pediatr Diabetes* 2000; **1**:181–5.
21. Rossetti L, Giaccari A, DeFronzo RA. Glucose toxicity. *Diabetes Care* 1990; **13**:610–30.
22. McGarry JD. Disordered metabolism in diabetes: have we underemphasized the fat component? *J Cell Biochem* 1994; **55**:29–38.
23. Kulkarni RN, Brüning JC, Winnay JN *et al*. Tissue-specific knock-out of the insulin receptor in pancreatic β cells creates an insulin secretory defect similar to that in type 2 diabetes. *Cell* 1999; **96**:329–39.
24. Garofano A, Czernichow P, Bréant B. In utero undernutrition impairs rat beta-cell development. *Diabetologia* 1997; **40**:1231–4.
25. Garofano A, Czernichow P, Bréant B. Effect of ageing on beta cell mass and function in rats malnourished during the perinatal period. *Diabetologia* 1999; **42**:711–18.
26. Yajnik CS, Fall CH, Vaidya U *et al*. Fetal growth and glucose and insulin metabolism in four-year-old Indian children. *Diabet Med* 1995; **12**:330–6.
27. Dabelea D, Pettitt DJ, Hanson RL *et al*. Birth weight, type 2 diabetes, and insulin resistance in Pima Indian children and young adults. *Diabetes Care* 1999; **22**:944–50.
28. Bavdekar A, Yajnik CS, Fall CH *et al*. Insulin resistance syndrome in 8-year-old Indian children: small at birth, big at 8 years, or both? *Diabetes* 1999; **48**:2422–9.
29. Hofman PL, Cutfield WS, Robinson EM *et al*. Insulin resistance in short children with intrauterine growth retardation. *J Clin Endocrinol Metab* 1997; **82**:402–6.
30. Wilkin TJ, Metcalf BS, Murphy MJ, Kirkby J, Jeffery AN, Voss LD. The relative contributions of birth weight, weight change, and current weight to insulin resistance in contemporary 5-year-olds: the EarlyBird Study. *Diabetes* 2002; **51**(12):3468–72.
31. Whincup PH, Cook DG, Adshead F *et al*. Childhood size is more strongly related than size at birth to glucose and insulin levels in 10–11-year-old children. *Diabetologia* 1997; **40**:319–26.
32. Hulman S, Kushner H, Katz S, Falkner B. Can cardiovascular risk be predicted by newborn, childhood, and adolescent body size? An examination of longitudinal data in urban African Americans. *J Pediatr* 1998; **132**:90–7.
33. Petersen S, Gotfredsen A, Ursin Knudsen F. Lean body mass in small for gestational age and appropriate for gestational age infants. *J Pediatr* 1988; **113**:886–9.
34. Jaquet D, Léger J, Lévy-Marchal, Oury JF *et al*. Ontogeny of leptin in human fetuses and newborns. Effect of intra-uterine growth retardation. *J Clin Endocrinol Metab* 1998; **83**:1243–6.
35. Enzi G, Zanardo V, Caretta F *et al*. Intrauterine growth and adipose tissue development. *Am J Clin Nutr* 1981; **34**:1785–90.
36. Albertsson-Wikland K, Wennergren G, Wennergren M *et al*. Longitudinal follow-up of growth in children born small for gestational age. *Acta Paediatr* 1993; **82**:438–43.

37. Jaquet D, Léger J, Tabone MD *et al.* High serum leptin concentrations during catch-up growth of children born with intra-uterine growth retardation. *J Clin Endocrinol Metab* 1999; **84**:1949–53.
38. Ravelli GP, Stein ZA, Susser MW. Obesity in young men after famine exposure in utero and early infancy. *N Engl J Med* 1976; **296**:349–53.
39. Ong KK, Ahmed ML, Emmett PM *et al.* Association between postnatal catch-up growth and obesity in childhood: prospective cohort study. *Br Med J* 2000; **320**:967–71.
40. Hediger ML, Overpeck MD, Kuczmarski RJ *et al.* Muscularity and fatness of infants and young children born small or large for gestational age. *Pediatrics* 1998; **102**:1–7.
41. Léger J, Limoni C, Collin D, Czernichow P. Prediction factors in the determination of final height in subjects born small for gestational age. *Pediatr Res* 1998; **43**:808–12.
42. Jaquet D, Gaboriau A, Czernichow P, Lévy-Marchal C. Relatively low serum leptin levels in adults born with intra-uterine growth retardation. *Int J Obes Relat Metab Disord* 2001; **25**:491–5.
43. Neel JV. Diabetes mellitus: a "thrifty" genotype rendered detrimental by "progress". *Am J Hum Genet* 1962; **14**:353–62.
44. Lucas A. Programming by early nutrition in man. In: *The childhood environment and adult disease*. CIBA Foundation Symposium 156. Chichester: Wiley, 1991: 38–55.
45. Lindsay RS, Dabelea D, Roumain J *et al.* Type 2 diabetes and low birth weight: the role of paternal inheritance in the association of low birth weight and diabetes. *Diabetes* 2000; **49**:445–9.
46. Hattersley AT, Tooke JE. The fetal insulin hypothesis: an alternative explanation of the association of low birthweight with diabetes and vascular disease. *Lancet* 1999; **353**:1789–92.
47. Ong KK, Phillips DI, Fall C *et al.* The insulin gene VNTR, type 2 diabetes and birth weight. *Nat Genet* 1999; **21**:262–3.
48. Vaessen N, Janssen JA, Heutink P *et al.* Association between genetic variation in the gene for insulin-like growth factor-I and low birthweight. *Lancet* 2002; **359**:1036–7.
49. Poulsen P, Vaag A, Beck-Nielsen H. Does zygosity influence the metabolic profile of twins? A population based cross sectional study. *Br Med J* 1999; **319**:151–4.
50. Poulsen P, Vaag AA, Kyvik KO *et al.* Low birth weight is associated with NIDDM in discordant monozygotic and dizygotic twin pairs. *Diabetologia* 1997; **40**:439–46.
51. Rizza RA, Mandarino LJ, Gerich JE. Cortisol-induced insulin resistance in man: impaired suppression of glucose production and stimulation of glucose utilization due to a postreceptor detect of insulin action. *J Clin Endocrinol Metab* 1982; **54**:131–8.
52. Hautanen A, Raikkonen K, Adlercreutz H. Associations between pituitary–adrenocortical function and abdominal obesity, hyperinsulinaemia and dyslipidaemia in normotensive males. *J Intern Med* 1997; **241**:451–61.
53. Pasquali R, Cantobelli S, Casimirri F *et al.* The hypothalamic–pituitary–adrenal axis in obese women with different patterns of body fat distribution. *J Clin Endocrinol Metab* 1993; **77**:341–6.

54. Phillips DI, Walker BR, Reynolds RM *et al*. Low birth weight predicts elevated plasma cortisol concentrations in adults from 3 populations. *Hypertension* 2000; **35**:1301–6.
55. Clark PM. Programming of the hypothalamo–pituitary–adrenal axis and the fetal origins of adult disease hypothesis. *Eur J Pediatr* 1998; **157**(Suppl 1):S7–10.
56. Clark PM, Hindmarsh PC, Shiell AW *et al*. Size at birth and adrenocortical function in childhood. *Clin Endocrinol* 1996; **45**:721–6.
57. Dahlgren J, Boguszewski M, Rosberg S, Albertsson-Wikland K. Adrenal steroid hormones in short children born small for gestational age. *Clin Endocrinol* 1998; **49**:353–61.
58. Ibañez L, Potau N, Virdis R *et al*. Postpubertal outcome in girls diagnosed with premature pubarche during childhood: increased frequency of functional ovarian hyperandrogenism. *J Clin Endocrinol Metab* 1993; **76**:1599–603.
59. Ibañez L, Potau N, Zampolli M *et al*. Hyperinsulinemia in postpubertal girls with a history of premature pubarche and functional ovarian hyperandrogenism. *J Clin Endocrinol Metab* 1996; **81**:1237–43.
60. Ibañez L, Potau N, Francois I, De Zegher F. Premature pubarche, hyperinsulinism and ovarian hyperandrogenism in girls: relation to reduced fetal growth. *J Clin Endocrinol Metab* 1998; **83**:3558–62.
61. Jaquet D, Leger J, Chevenne D, Czernichow P, Levy-Marchal C. Intrauterine growth retardation predisposes to insulin resistance but not to hyperandrogenism in young women. *J Clin Endocrinol Metab* 1999; **84**:3945–9.
62. Cresswell JL, Barker DJP, Osmond C *et al*. Fetal growth, length of gestation, and polycystic ovaries in adult life. *Lancet* 1997; **350**:1131–5.

chapter 8

Clinical manifestations of the metabolic syndrome and type 2 diabetes in childhood and adolescence

Jill Hamilton and Denis Daneman

Introduction

The complex association of impaired glucose metabolism (including insulin resistance, glucose intolerance, or type 2 diabetes), obesity (particularly visceral adiposity), hyperlipidemia, and hypertension has been well documented in adults. Initially termed 'syndrome X' by Reaven, this clustering of factors has subsequently been known as the metabolic syndrome, dysmetabolic syndrome, or insulin resistance syndrome.[1,2] Recently, the World Health Organization proposed a unifying definition for the metabolic syndrome in adults (Table 8.1). Irrespective of the term applied to this disorder, the health and economic burden to society is enormous, and will continue to escalate as the prevalence of type 2 diabetes and the metabolic syndrome rises worldwide.

There is no doubt that the metabolic syndrome has its roots in early life.[3] Adaptations to glucose metabolism and 'programming' for later development of insulin resistance may even begin in utero (see Chapter 7). The global increase in type 2 diabetes includes older children and adolescents and, as in adults, this closely parallels the rising trend of obesity.[4–6] Despite predictions of an epidemic of type 2 diabetes in young individuals,

Table 8.1 Definition of the metabolic syndrome in adults[1]

Insulin resistance, impaired glucose tolerance or type 2 diabetes plus two of:

Obesity	WHR, females>0.85, males >0.9
	and/or BMI >30 kg/m²
Hypertension	BP ≥ 160/90 mmHg
Dyslipidemia	Triglycerides ≥ 1.7 mmol/l and/or HDL cholesterol
	females < 1.0, males < 0.9 mmol/l
Microalbuminuria	Albumin excretion rate ≥ 20 μg/min
	or albumin:creatinine ratio ≥ 20 mg/g

WHR = waist:hip ratio, BP = blood pressure, HDL = high-density lipoprotein.

there is, in fact, scant literature in this population. This is likely due in part to the relatively recent increased frequency of this condition in young people. The first few reports of the appearance of type 2 diabetes in Native American and Canadian children appeared about 20 years ago and only in the past 5–10 years have other groups reported their experiences in Japanese, North American white, African-American, and Hispanic children.[7] In this chapter, we review the metabolic syndrome and type 2 diabetes in childhood and adolescence, emphasizing recognizable risk factors and the variable clinical manifestations of this spectrum of disorders.

Risk factors and clinical features

Obesity

There is a strong association of type 2 diabetes and obesity: the globally rising prevalence of obesity indicates that there will inevitably be more youth diagnosed with this type of diabetes.[8] Sedentary lifestyle and increased availability of large-quantity, densely caloric foods are thought to be responsible for the staggering increase in childhood obesity, although the relative contributions of the two remain uncertain.[9] A report from the National Health and Nutrition Examination Survey (NHANES) determined that the prevalence of overweight children had doubled over a 15-year period between 1980 and 1994.[10] Based on normative data collected from 1963–70, NHANES in 1994 revealed that 22% of children were 'at risk of overweight' – defined as body mass index (BMI) 85–95th centile – and 10.9% were 'overweight' (BMI > 95th centile).[4] The highest overweight prevalence rates occurred in African-American girls and Mexican-American boys. In addition, the Bogalusa Heart Study, a 20-year longitudinal study which tracked over 11,500 children aged 5–17 years at recruitment, has shown a clear upward trend in weight, equivalent to a 0.2 kg increase in body weight/year at any given age.[11]

The Bogalusa Heart Study has also shown that high childhood BMI is a significant predictor of the metabolic syndrome during adulthood.[12] Investigators followed subjects from childhood for 11.6 ± 3.4 years to assess the appearance of various aspects of the metabolic syndrome and atherosclerotic heart disease. They demonstrated that 77% of the 186 overweight children remained obese as adults, whereas only 7% of 1317 normal-weight children became obese adults.[13] They did not, however, detect an independent relationship of childhood obesity with adult development of the metabolic syndrome after adjustment for adult obesity. The entire cohort of adults was analyzed by separation of individual risk factors (BMI, fasting insulin, systolic or mean blood pressure, and total cholesterol : HDL cholesterol ratio or triglyceride : HDL ratio) into quartiles. The proportion of adults with clustering of all four risk factors increased across childhood BMI. The study concluded that childhood obesity is an important predictor of adult obesity and the metabolic syndrome. Due to strong tracking of obesity into adulthood, it is difficult to tease out the significance of the age of obesity onset in relation to subsequent severity of obesity, risk factor levels, or other co-morbidities such as type 2 diabetes and atherosclerotic heart disease in adulthood.

Early onset of obesity has been shown to be a risk factor for development of type 2 diabetes in childhood.[14] There are extensive data that obesity, and in particular, visceral adiposity, is strongly linked to insulin resistance in both prepubertal and pubertal children.[15–18] Obesity is a very common finding in youth with type 2 diabetes. Although the definition of obesity varies between reports, the range of mean BMI in children with type 2 diabetes has been reported to be between 29 and 38 kg/m^2, with the vast majority above the 85th percentile for age and sex norms[6,14,19,20] (Table 8.2). Furthermore, in selected screening of very obese children and teens, impaired glucose tolerance has been detected in 4–25%.[21,22]

Ethnicity

Certain ethnic groups are over-represented in the reported clinic experiences of type 2 diabetes in youth. Specifically, African-American, Hispanic, Asian, and Native American children are much more likely to develop type 2 diabetes during childhood than are their white American peers.[6] In Japan, the incidence of type 2 diabetes in children has also increased dramatically and is seven times more common than type 1 diabetes in the adolescent age range (13.9 vs 2.0 per 100,000).[23,24] We recently surveyed our diabetes population at the Hospital for Sick Children (HSC) in Toronto, Canada. Of 1020 children with diabetes attending our diabetes clinic, 40 (4%) were identified as having type 2 diabetes. Although Toronto is heralded as one of the most multicultural cities in the world, with visible minorities comprising over 30% of the population, we found over-representation of certain minority ethnic groups relative to the regional population among our youth with type 2 diabetes. Specifically, 26% were of African/Carribean descent, 47% South or East Asian, 19% Caucasian, 5% Hispanic, and 3% other.

Sinha *et al.*[21] examined the prevalence of impaired glucose tolerance and type 2 diabetes in a selected population of obese children and reported a surprisingly high rate of glucose intolerance in all ethnic groups. They screened 167 (97 non-Hispanic white, 38 non-Hispanic black, 32 Hispanic) asymptomatic obese children (BMI > 95th centile for age and gender) using an oral glucose tolerance test and found impaired glucose tolerance in 25%. Of these, 51% were white, 30% black, and 19% Hispanic. All four of the individuals with diagnosed type 2 diabetes were, however, of non-Hispanic black or Hispanic origin. This may suggest that certain prediabetic metabolic abnormalities (e.g. impaired glucose tolerance) are present equally across all ethnic groups but that type 2 diabetes develops earlier in high-risk ethnic groups. This may be related to a higher frequency of obesity in the African-American

Table 8.2 Clinical characteristics of youth with type 2 diabetes (adapted from Dabelea et al.[19] and Fagot-Campagna et al.[6])

Year	Location	Number of cases	AA (%)	H (%)	C (%)	FN/NA (%)	Mean age at diagnosis	Female/male ratio	Mean BMI (kg/m²)	Family history T2DM (%)
1992	Manitoba[76]	20	–	–	–	100	12	4.0	26	100
1996	Sioux Lookout, ON[30]	15	–	–	–	100	12	14	29	93
	Cincinnati, OH[59]	54	69	–	31	–	14	1.7	38	85
1997	Charleston, SC[73]	39	100	–	–	–	13	1.3	30	95
	Little Rock, AR[78]	50	74	2	24	–	14	1.6	35	–
1998	San Diego, CA[79]	18	11	67	17	–	13	2.0	27	87
	San Antonio, TX[44]	101	–	83	–	–	13	3.0	–	74
	Chicago, IL[81]	160	75	25	–	–	14	1.7	33	50
	Ventura, CA[80]	21	–	100	–	–	14	0.8	33	100
	Gila River, AZ[27]	100	–	–	–	100	16	1.7	35	–
	Hartford, CT[20]	17	29	42	–	–	–	1.8	36	–
2002	Brooklyn, NY[49]	37	86	11	3	–	–	–	32	–
	Houston, TX[82]	25	28	60	7	–	13	1.3	a	100
	Toronto, Ont[b]	40	26	5	19	2.5	14	1.7	32	94

a All > 85th centile for age and gender.
b Unpublished data.
AA = African-American, H = Hispanic, C = Caucasian, FN/NA = First Nation, Native American, BMI = body mass index, T2DM = type 2 diabetes mellitus.

and Native American populations during childhood.[4,25–27] There may also be inherent differences in metabolism. Physiologic data from Arslanian and others demonstrate a lower insulin sensitivity and higher fasting insulin level in prepubertal and pubertal African-American children compared to age, sex, puberty, and BMI matched Caucasian children.[28] In all probability, a combination of both environmental (physical activity level, nutrient intake) and genetic factors combine to account for these variations in the rate of type 2 diabetes in different ethnic populations.

Of note is that the vast majority of studies, which include referral bias with data collected from diabetes clinic populations, are not population-based. Detailed prevalence studies have been performed in Native-North American children[26,29,30] and a population prevalence study was carried out in Bangladesh.[85] Until larger prevalence studies are completed in more diverse populations, it will remain impossible to define relative risk rates for different ethnic groups. An additional challenge is that a rapidly rising incidence of obesity will modify the rate of appearance of type 2 diabetes, rendering accurate ascertainment difficult.

Family history

In most youth with type 2 diabetes, there are likely to be several family members previously diagnosed with this condition. Studies of African-American, Caucasian, Hispanic, and American Indian or First Nation youth document a first- or second-degree relative with type 2 diabetes in 50–100% of families (Table 8.2).[6,19] Furthermore, in a study of 11 children with type 2 diabetes, their first-degree relatives were also quite likely to be obese, sedentary, and eat high-fat, low-fibre food.[31] A study that retrospectively assessed 854 children's weights to adulthood examined the relationship between parent and child obesity and how this tracks over time.[32] Parental obesity more than doubled the risk of adult obesity among children under 10 years of age. These data imply that the occurrence of early-onset type 2 diabetes is influenced by two groups of factors – similarities in lifestyle within the family unit, creating an environmental trigger in the genetically at risk.

Age of diagnosis

The majority of youth with type 2 diabetes are diagnosed following the onset of puberty (Table 8.2). The mean age in most reports varies between 12 and 14 years of age.[6] In the Pima Indian and Ojibway-Cree populations there have been exceptional reports of type 2 diabetes in prepubertal children, the youngest being 4 years of age at diagnosis.[26,29] In the 40 children with type 2 diabetes attending our clinic, the mean age of diagnosis was 13.9 years (range 9–18 years).

There have been numerous physiologic studies that demonstrate decreased insulin sensitivity during puberty in children[33–35] (see Chapter 10). Insulin resistance increases in early puberty (Tanner 2), peaks in mid-puberty (Tanner 3), with improvement in late puberty (Tanner 4–5). Puberty-related insulin resistance is believed to be secondary to the effects of increased growth hormone secretion.[35] Normally, decreased pubertal insulin sensitivity is compensated for by increased insulin secretion.[34] However, in the individual with multiple risk factors for type 2 diabetes who is already hyperinsulinemic, puberty may be the final trigger that leads to metabolic decompensation and impaired glucose tolerance.

Female gender and polycystic ovary syndrome (PCOS)

With the exception of one report of equal sex distribution, there is a female preponderance among youth with type 2 diabetes, with female-to-male ratios of 1.3–1.8 reported (Table 8.2).[6,19] In our clinic, 63% of patients are female (female-to-male ratio 1.7). The reason for the female preponderance is unclear, although some investigators have demonstrated a greater degree of insulin resistance in girls than in boys at all stages of puberty.[35,36]

PCOS is defined as hyperandrogenism with chronic anovulation and is associated with oligo- or amenorrhea, hirsutism, and hyperinsulinism.[37] In adult women with PCOS, impaired glucose tolerance and type 2 diabetes are common and substantially more so than in age- and weight-matched populations of women without PCOS.[38,39] Recently, studies in postpubertal adolescents confirmed that insulin resistance is more severe in girls with PCOS compared with their obese but nonhyperandrogenic peers.[40,41] There are no large prevalence studies of impaired glucose tolerance in adolescents with PCOS, although in one report of 27 adolescents referred for PCOS, impaired glucose tolerance was detected in 30% and unrecognized diabetes in one individual.[42] Importantly, the abnormalities in glucose metabolism were detected by oral glucose tolerance testing and not by fasting blood glucose. Data about frequency of PCOS in youth with type 2 diabetes are limited. We have found PCOS in 16% (4/25) of our female patients with type 2 diabetes.

Acanthosis nigricans

Acanthosis nigricans (AN) refers to velvety, thickened, hyperpigmented lesions that appear in skinfold areas such as the nape of the neck, axillae, antecubital fossae, and groin (Figure 8.1). Histologically, papillomatosis and hyperkeratosis are present and are believed to be secondary

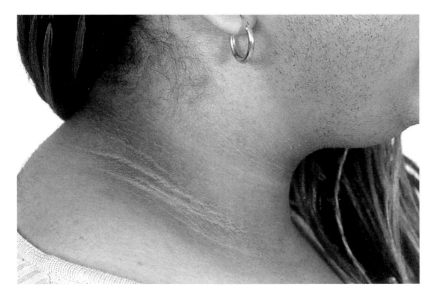

Figure 8.1 *Fifteen-year-old female with type 2 diabetes and polycystic ovarian syndrome. Note significant acanthosis nigricans in the neck region and severe hirsutism.*

to local stimulation of unidentified cutaneous growth factors by insulin.[43] AN is common in African-American, Native American, and First Nation individuals but has also been reported in Hispanic, South and East Asian, and Caucasian children.[43,44] It is seen frequently in obese children with glucose intolerance, is easy to note on routine clinical examination, and is an excellent clinical marker of insulin resistance.

A retrospective chart review of 33 children with AN (19% African-American, 67% Hispanic, and 7% Caucasian) found that 94% had a BMI above the 95th centile, 82% had a first- or second-degree relative with type 2 diabetes, 22% PCOS, 24% impaired glucose tolerance, and 3% type 2 diabetes.[45] A recent population-based screening study of middle school students demonstrated AN in 19% of students.[46] The presence of AN was associated with obesity and hyperinsulinism.

AN has been found in 40–90% of youth with type 2 diabetes.[6,19] Although AN is clearly associated with type 2 diabetes and impaired glucose tolerance, it may actually be a marker more specific for obesity than insulin resistance. A study in 114 children compared insulin resistance as measured by hyperglycemic clamp with adiposity measured by dual-energy X-ray absorptiometry.[47] Although children with AN were more insulin resistant than those without AN, this was no longer significant following adjustment for differences in body fat. BMI alone was found to be a better predictor of insulin resistance than AN.

Dyslipidemia and other risk factors for atherogenesis

Cardiovascular disease is responsible for 80% of deaths in adults with type 2 diabetes with age-adjusted relative risk three times higher than in the general population.[48] Factors related to cardiovascular disease described by the metabolic syndrome include insulin resistance, hypertension, dyslipidemia, hypercoagulability, impaired fibrinolysis, and proinflammatory state interactions.[49] The typical 'atherogenic' dyslipidemia consists of elevated triglycerides with small low-density lipoprotein (LDL) particles and low HDL cholesterol.[50]

In the non-diabetic pediatric population, obesity has been associated with the clustering of other features of the metabolic syndrome, including systolic hypertension, dyslipidemia, and insulin resistance.[51–54] Investigators have also demonstrated markers of insulin resistance such as elevated C-reactive protein and plasminogen activator inhibitor-1 (PAI-1) in obese children.[55–57] Thus, similar associations of factors related to the metabolic syndrome that are well documented in adults also appear to be present in children, although the extent of these associations will vary depending on factors such as age and pubertal status.

It is difficult to relate risk factors for the metabolic syndrome in childhood to adult cardiovascular disease outcome due to the long follow-up periods and large patient populations required. Few studies have been able to quantitate asymptomatic atherosclerosis in relation to the metabolic syndrome during youth. The Pathobiological Determinants of Atherosclerosis in Youth (PDAY) Research Group has performed autopsies on over 3000 individuals aged 15–34 years who died of accidental/ traumatic causes.[58] They obtained pathologic information in a standardized fashion, and found a close link between atherosclerotic changes and increased BMI, adiposity, elevated total cholesterol and lowered HDL cholesterol levels, tobacco smoke exposure, hypertension, and chronic hyperglycemia. Similarly, autopsies were performed on 93 young people (age 2–39 years) from the Bogalusa Heart Study who had died primarily from trauma. The data confirmed that the presence of risk factors associated with the metabolic syndrome in childhood is predictive of later morbidity.

There is information available on the prevalence of hypertension and hyperlipidemia in children with type 2 diabetes. In a cohort of Pima Indian children aged 5–19 years, 4092 (86.4%) had normal glucose tolerance, 546 (11.5%) impaired glucose tolerance, and 100 (2.1%) type 2 diabetes. The prevalence of hypertension (defined as blood pressure > 140/90 mmHg) was 5, 10, and 18%, respectively, and hypercholesterolemia (cholesterol > 200 mg/dl) 6, 6, and 7%.[27] In a group of 54 children with type 2 diabetes from Cincinnati, 17% had hypertension at diagnosis and 4% hypertriglyceridemia.[59] In African-American youth with type 2 diabetes presenting in ketoacidosis, 42% had previously diagnosed hypertension.[60] Among 40 African-American children with type 2 diabetes (mean age 15.3 years, BMI 34.4 kg/m^2, HbA$_{1c}$ 9.8%) from New York City, 44% had elevated triglycerides, 15% low HDL, and high LDL, defined as >90th centile for age and sex for triglyceride and LDL and less than 10th centile for HDL.[61]

Nonalcoholic steatohepatitis (NASH)

NASH has been recognized for 20 years but has only recently been linked to type 2 diabetes and, in particular, the metabolic syndrome.[62] It is characterized by chronic elevation of hepatic transaminases and histologic changes consistent with alcoholic hepatitis in the absence of alcohol intake and after secondary causes of hepatitis have been excluded.[63] Adult patients with NASH have many characteristics of the metabolic syndrome with hyperlipidemia, visceral obesity, insulin resistance, type 2 diabetes, and hypertension.[64–66]

Originally believed to be a benign condition, NASH is now recognized as a cause of progressive liver disease which may lead to fibrotic cirrhosis and hepatic failure.[62] In the Verona Diabetes Study, a population-based study in Italy, the standardized mortality ratio for hepatic cirrhosis was 2.52 (CI 1.96–3.20) in a group of adults with type 2 diabetes compared with the general population.[67] The inflammatory state and subsequent oxidative stress associated with hyperinsulinism and the metabolic syndrome may be the underlying cause of hepatocellular damage in NASH.[68]

In children, elevated hepatic transaminases have been reported in approximately 25% of Japanese and Italian obese children examined during screening.[69,70] In a prospective series of 36 children aged 4–16 years with NASH from the Hospital for Sick Children in Toronto, 30 (83%) were obese, 18 (50%) had hyperlipidemia, 13 (36%) had acanthosis nigricans, and 4 (11%) were diagnosed with or developed type 2 diabetes during childhood.[71] One 10-year-old patient without type 2 diabetes in this group had established cirrhosis at diagnosis.

The frequency of NASH in youth with type 2 diabetes has not been studied. Although the long-term prognosis in children is unclear, the associated morbidity in adults makes it important to document this disease carefully in the young. Weight loss and/or treatment with antioxidants such as vitamin E have been shown in uncontrolled trials to lower transaminase levels and may also be beneficial therapy in young people with NASH.[72]

Presentation of type 2 diabetes in childhood

Type 2 diabetes may present in typical or atypical fashion. The 'typical' patient is an obese female adolescent, belonging to a high-risk ethnic group, with a positive family history for type 2 diabetes and who may have a history of menstrual irregularities suggestive of PCOS. She has a history of slow-onset (months) of increasing thirst, polyuria, and nocturia, with a variable degree of weight loss. Fasting and postprandial glucose levels are in the diabetic range, ketones are absent, tests for islet cell antibodies and anti-GAD antibodies are negative, and C-peptide levels are measurable and often high (at least after the hyperglycemia has been controlled).

Although this description applies to the 'typical' patient, there is great heterogeneity in the appearance of type 2 diabetes, which can make the diagnosis quite challenging. Information was available on 47 children with type 2 diabetes from Cincinnati.[59] Only 19% presented with the classic symptoms of polyuria, polydipsia, and weight loss, whereas 32% were identified by urinalysis during a routine examination. Twenty four percent of girls had vaginal monilial infection as the primary complaint and the remainder were found to have type 2 diabetes during investigation for a variety of complaints, including obesity, infection, dysuria, enuresis, and abdominal pain.

Type 2 diabetes in youth, as in adults, may have an indolent presentation and be asymptomatic. Large prevalence studies have not been performed; however, in two series studying very high-risk individuals (obese with multiethnic background and First Nation), asymptomatic diabetes was found in 3.6% of adolescents.[21,26] The American Diabetes Association has recommended testing children from age 10 years or at onset of puberty (if less than 10 years) every 2 years with fasting plasma glucose if they are overweight and have any two of the following risk factors: family history type 2 diabetes, high risk ethnicity, signs of insulin resistance (acanthosis nigricans, hypertension, dyslipidemia, PCOS) (see Chapter 1). Interestingly, the study by Sinha *et al.*[21] published following these recommendations, determined that the 2-h glucose level following the oral glucose tolerance test (OGTT) was much more sensitive in diagnosing both impaired glucose tolerance (IGT) and diabetes than fasting glucose levels. Of the 37 children with IGT, none would have been detected by fasting glucose alone and all of the 4 subjects diagnosed with type 2 diabetes by OGTT would have been misclassified as IFG by fasting glucose measurement. This finding was duplicated in a study examining adolescent girls with PCOS and IGT – only the OGTT identified those with glucose intolerance.[42] This requires further study and may indicate that different screening methods are required in the pediatric population.

Some youth with type 2 diabetes have a more acute onset with severe symptoms, including: weight loss and dehydration, with significantly elevated blood glucose concentration, and ketonuria or frank ketoacidosis. Many are African-American children and this presentation has sometimes been referred to as 'flatbush diabetes' or 'atypical diabetes in African-Americans (ADM)'.[49,60,73,74] In the Cincinnati series of islet cell antibody negative individuals, 42% of the 28 African-American patients presented with ketonuria, and 25% with ketoacidosis, whereas none of the 12 white adolescents with type 2 diabetes had ketonuria either at diagnosis or during follow-up.[60] Another group in Charleston, South Carolina, reported on 29 African-American type 2 patients, defined as having negative ICA and GAD antibodies and elevated fasting C-peptide levels.[73] Within this group, 16 (55%) had experienced ketosis and 11 (38%) had been hospitalized for ketoacidosis. In both studies, there was no difference between the age, BMI, or sex distribution of patients with and without ketones at presentation.

Arslanian and others have documented metabolic differences in glucose homeostasis in non-diabetic African-American children compared with their peers (see Chapter 6). This includes increased insulin resistance at all ages, increased baseline insulin, and increased insulin secretion in response to acute glucose elevation compared to age, weight, and pubertal stage matched Caucasian children.[28] In addition, African-American youth with type 2 diabetes, similar to adults with type 2 diabetes, have documented beta-cell decompensation with inappropriately low insulin secretion in response to a glucose challenge.[75] This beta-cell dysfunction may be related in part to acute glucose toxicity, as reports of weaning or discontinuing insulin with maintenance of good glycemic control exist.[75] Although ketonuria has been reported most frequently in African-American youth, there is documentation of ketoacidosis across all ethnic groups.[49,73,76–81] Clearly, the presence of ketones can make the distinction between type 1 and type 2 diabetes more difficult (see Chapter 1).

Maturity onset diabetes of youth (MODY) represents another group of conditions with diabetes presenting in childhood and distinct from classical type 2 diabetes. MODY may be discovered either incidentally or with mild symptoms of polyuria/polydipsia. MODY is a group of disorders characterized by an autosomal dominant inheritance of diabetes mellitus in childhood or early adulthood (see also Chapter 11).[82] MODY can be divided into 6 subgroups based on the genetic mutations, with the most common being the glucokinase (MODY2) and HNF-1α (MODY3) genes.[83] In general, individuals with MODY1 or 3 are nonobese Caucasian individuals who present with nonketotic, mild, or asymptomatic hyperglycemia.[74,84]

In summary, the diagnosis of type 2 diabetes is often not clear-cut when the presenting symptoms (or lack thereof) overlap with type 1 diabetes, autosomal dominant MODY, or atypical diabetes mellitus with ketones. Certain tests (islet cell and antiGAD antibodies, C-peptide level, genetic testing for MODY) may be helpful, but often the diagnosis only becomes apparent over time with the observed response to therapy.

Conclusion

The rapid rise in obesity is associated with both an increasing prevalence of type 2 diabetes throughout the world and a decreasing age of onset of the condition. The vast majority of reports of type 2 diabetes in youth have been clinic-based. Research efforts at the population level are required not only to determine the frequency of type 2 diabetes but also to assess the importance of identifiable risk factors and chart the early course of the disorder.

There is clearly a clustering of risk factors for the metabolic syndrome in childhood as in adults. What is not known is the extent of some of these abnormalities, such as hypertension and dyslipidemia, in youth with type 2 diabetes. Furthermore, the relationship between type 2 diabetes in youth with other disorders such as PCOS and NASH remains to be elucidated. There is no doubt that this will continue to be an important and productive area for research in the years to come. However, it is the prevention and treatment of obesity and type 2 diabetes in youth that provide the most daunting challenges to our health care systems.

References

1. Alberti KG, Zimmet PZ. Definition, diagnosis and classification of diabetes mellitus and its complications. Part 1: diagnosis and classification of diabetes mellitus provisional report of a WHO consultation. *Diabet Med* 1998; **15**(7):539–53.
2. Reaven GM. Role on insulin resistance in human disease. *Diabetes* 1988; **37**:1595–607.
3. Ong KK, Dunger DB. Perinatal growth failure: the road to obesity, insulin resistance and cardiovascular disease in adults. *Best Pract Res Clin Endocrinol Metab* 2002; **16**(2):191–207.
4. Troiano RP, Flegal KM, Kuczmarski RJ. Overweight prevalence and trends for children and adolescents. *Arch Pediatr Adolesc Med* 1995; **149**:1085–91.
5. Freedman DS, Srinivasan SR, Valdez RA, Williamson DF, Berenson GS. Secular increases in relative weight and adiposity among children over two decades: the Bogalusa Heart Study. *Pediatrics* 1997; **99**:420–6.
6. Fagot-Campagna A, Pettitt DJ, Engelgau MM *et al*. Type 2 diabetes among North American children and adolescents: an epidemiologic review and a public health perspective. *J Pediatr* 2000; **136**(5):664–72.
7. Fagot-Campagna A. Emergence of type 2 diabetes mellitus in children: epidemiological evidence. *J Pediatr Endocrinol* 2000; **13**(suppl 6):1395–402.
8. Deckelbaum RJ, Williams CL. Childhood obesity: the health issue. *Obesity Res* 2001; **9**(suppl 4):239–43S.
9. Zimmet P, Alberti KG, Shaw J. Global and societal implications of the diabetes epidemic. *Nature* 2001; **414**(6865):782–7.
10. Troiano RP, Flegal KM. Overweight children and adolescents: description, epidemiology and demographics. *Pediatrics* 1998; **101**:497–504.
11. Freedman DS, Srinivasan SR, Valdez RA, Williamson DF, Berenson GS. Secular increases in relative weight and adiposity among children over two decades: the Bogalusa Heart Study. *Pediatrics* 1997; **99**(3):420–6.
12. Srinivasan SR, Myers L, Berenson GS. Predictability of childhood adiposity and insulin for developing insulin resistance syndrome (syndrome X) in young adulthood: the Bogalusa Heart Study. *Diabetes* 2002; **51**(1):204–9.
13. Freedman DS, Khan LK, Dietz WH, Srinivasan SR, Berenson GS. Relationship of childhood obesity to coronary heart disease risk factors in adulthood: the Bogalusa Heart Study. *Pediatrics* 2001; **108**(3):712–18.

14. American Diabetes Association. Consensus statement: Type 2 diabetes in children and adolescents. *Diabetes Care* 2000; **23**(3):381–9.
15. Arslanian S, Suprasongsin C. Insulin sensitivity, lipids, and body composition in childhood: is "syndrome X" present? *J Clin Endocrinol Metabol* 1996; **81**(3):1058–62.
16. Caprio S, Hyman LD, Limb C *et al.* Central adiposity and its metabolic correlates in obese adolescent girls. *Am J Physiol* 1995; **269**(1 Pt 1):E118–26.
17. Caprio S, Bronson M, Sherwin RS, Rife F, Tamborlane WV. Co-existence of severe insulin resistance and hyperinsulinaemia in pre-adolescent obese children. *Diabetologia* 1996; **39**(12):1489–97.
18. Steinberger J, Moorehead C, Katch V, Rocchini AP. Relationship between insulin resistance and abnormal lipid profile in obese adolescents. *J Pediatr* 1995; **126**(5 Pt 1):690–5.
19. Dabelea D, Pettitt DJ, Jones KL, Arslanian SA. Type 2 diabetes mellitus in minority children and adolescents. An emerging problem. *Endocrinol Metabol Clin N Am* 1999; **28**(4):709–29, viii.
20. Langshur S, Onyirimba M, Estrada E. Type 2 diabetes in childhood, one year follow-up on insulin treatment in comparison with children with type 1 diabetes. *Diabetes* 1998; **47**(suppl 1):A83.
21. Sinha R, Fisch G, Teague B *et al.* Prevalence of impaired glucose tolerance among children and adolescents with marked obesity. *N Engl J Med* 2002; **346**(11):802–10.
22. Sinha R, Fisch G, Teague B *et al.* Impaired glucose tolerance in children and adolescents – correspondence. *N Engl J Med* 2002; **347**(4):290–2.
23. Kitagawa T, Owada M, Urakami T, Tajima N. Epidemiology of type 1 (insulin-dependent) and type 2 (non-insulin-dependent) diabetes mellitus in Japanese children. *Diabetes Res Clin Pract* – supplement. 1994; **24**(suppl):S7–13.
24. Kitagawa T, Owada M, Urakami T, Yamauchi K. Increased incidence of non-insulin dependent diabetes mellitus among Japanese schoolchildren correlates with an increased intake of animal protein and fat. *Clin Pediatr* 1998; **37**(2):111–15.
25. Jackson MY. Height, weight, and body mass index of American Indian school-children. *J Am Diet Assoc* 1993; **93**:1136–40.
26. Dean HJ, Young TK, Flett B, Wood-Steinman P. Screening for non-type 2 diabetes in aboriginal children in northern Canada (letter). *Lancet* 1998; **352**:1523–4.
27. Fagot-Campagna A, Knowler WC, Pettitt DJ. Type 2 diabetes in Pima Indian children: cardiovascular risk factors at diagnosis and 10 years later. *Diabetes* 1998; **47** (suppl 1):A155.
28. Arslanian S. Insulin secretion and sensitivity in healthy African-American vs American white children. *Clin Pediatr* 1998; **37**(2):81–8.
29. Dabelea D, Hanson RL, Bennett PH, Roumain J, Knowler WC, Pettitt DJ. Increasing prevalence of Type II diabetes in American Indian children. *Diabetologia* 1998; **41**(8):904–10.
30. Harris SB, Perkins BA, Whalen-Brough E. Non-insulin dependent diabetes mellitus among First Nations children. *Can Fam Phys* 1996; **42**:869–76.
31. Pinhas-Hamiel O, Standiford D, Hamiel D, Dolan LM, Cohen R, Zeitler PS. The type 2 family: a setting for development and treatment of adolescent type 2 diabetes mellitus. *Arch Pediatr Adolesc Med* 1999; **153**(10):1063–7.

32. Whitaker RC, Wright JA, Pepe MS, Seidel KD, Dietz WH. Predicting obesity in young adulthood from childhood and parental obesity. *N Engl J Med* 1997; **337**(13):869–73.
33. Amiel SA, Sherwin RS, Simonson DC, Lauritano AA, Tamborlane WV. Impaired insulin action in puberty. A contributing factor to poor control in adolescents with diabetes. *N Engl J Med* 1986; **315**(4):215–19.
34. Caprio S. Insulin: the other anabolic hormone of puberty. *Acta Paediatrica* 1999; **88**(433):84–7.
35. Moran A, Jacobs DR, Steinberger J *et al*. Insulin resistance during puberty. Results from clamp studies in 357 children. *Diabetes* 1999; **48**:2039–44.
36. Arslanian SA, Heil BV, Becker DJ, Drash AL. Sexual dimorphism in insulin sensitivity in adolescents with insulin-dependent diabetes mellitus. *J Clin Endocrinol Metabol* 1991; **72**(4):920–6.
37. Dunaif A, Thomas A. Current concepts in the polycystic ovary syndrome. *Ann Rev Med* 2001; **52**:401–19.
38. Ehrmann DA, Barnes RB, Rosenfield RL, Cavaghan MK, Imperial J. Prevalence of impaired glucose tolerance and diabetes in women with polycystic ovary syndrome. *Diabetes Care* 1999; **22**(1):141–6.
39. Legro RS, Kunselman AR, Dodson WC, Dunaif A. Prevalence and predictors of risk for type 2 diabetes mellitus and impaired glucose tolerance in polycystic ovary syndrome: a prospective, controlled study in 254 affected women. *J Clin Endocrinol Metabol* 1999; **84**(1):165–9.
40. Mauras N, Welch S, Rini A, Haymond MW. Ovarian hyperandrogenism is associated with insulin resistance to both peripheral carbohydrate and whole-body protein metabolism in postpubertal young females: a metabolic study. *J Clin Endocrinol Metabol* 1998; **83**(6):1900–5.
41. Lewy VD, Danadian K, Witchel SF, Arslanian S. Early metabolic abnormalities in adolescent girls with polycystic ovarian syndrome. *J Pediatrics* 2001; **138**(1):38–44.
42. Palmert MR, Gordon CM, Kartashov AI, Legro RS, Emans SJ, Dunaif A. Screening for abnormal glucose tolerance in adolescents with polycystic ovary syndrome. *J Clin Endocrinol Metabol* 2002; **87**(3):1017–23.
43. Stuart CA, Driscoll MS, Lundquist KF, Gilkison CR, Shaheb S, Smith MM. Acanthosis nigricans. *J Bas Clin Physiol Pharmacol* 1998; **9**(2–4): 407–18.
44. Hale DE, Danney MM. Non-insulin dependent diabetes in Hispanic youth (Type 2Y). *Diabetes* 1998; **47**(suppl 1):A82.
45. Brickman WJ, Howard JC, Metzger BE. Abnormal glucose tolerance in children with acanthosis nigricans: a chart review. *Diabetes* 2002; **51**(suppl 2):A429.
46. Mukhtar Q, Cleverley G, Voorhees RE, McGrath JW. Prevalence of acanthosis nigricans and its association with hyperinsulinemia in New Mexico adolescents. *J Adolesc Health* 2001; **28**(5):372–6.
47. Nguyen TT, Keil MF, Russell DL *et al*. Relation of acanthosis nigricans to hyperinsulinemia and insulin sensitivity in overweight African American and white children. *J Pediatr* 2001; **138**(4):474–80.
48. Haffner SM, Lehto S, Ronnemaa T, Pyorala K, Laakso M. Mortality from coronary heart disease in subjects with type 2 diabetes and in nondiabetic subjects with and without prior myocardial infarction. *N Engl J Med* 1998; **339**(4):229–34.

49. Umpaichitra V, Banerji M, Castells S. Autoantibodies in children with type 2 diabetes mellitus. *J Pediatr Endocrinol Metabol* 2002; **15**(suppl 1):S25–30.
50. Grundy SM. Obesity, metabolic syndrome, and coronary atherosclerosis. *Circulation* 2002; **105**(23):2696–8.
51. Gidding SS, Bao W, Srinivasan SR, Berenson GS. Effects of secular trends in obesity on coronary risk factors in children: the Bogalusa Heart Study. *J Pediatr* 1995; **127**(6):868–74.
52. Perrone J, Hollander JE, De Roos F. Cardiovascular risk factors and atherosclerosis in children and young adults. *N Engl J Med* 1998; **339**(15):1083–4.
53. Sinaiko AR, Donahue RP, Jacobs DR Jr, Prineas RJ. Relation of weight and rate of increase in weight during childhood and adolescence to body size, blood pressure, fasting insulin, and lipids in young adults. The Minneapolis Children's Blood Pressure Study. *Circulation* 1999; **99**(11):1471–6.
54. Sinaiko AR, Steinberger J, Moran A, Prineas RJ, Jacobs DR Jr. Relation of insulin resistance to blood pressure in childhood. *J Hypertension* 2002; **20**(3):509–17.
55. Cook DG, Mendall MA, Whincup PH et al. C-reactive protein concentration in children: relationship to adiposity and other cardiovascular risk factors. *Atherosclerosis* 2000; **149**(1):139–50.
56. Ford ES, Galuska DA, Gillespie C, Will JC, Giles WH, Dietz WH. C-reactive protein and body mass index in children: findings from the Third National Health and Nutrition Examination Survey, 1988–1994. *J Pediatr* 2001; **138**(4):486–92.
57. Sudi K, Gallistl S, Payerl D et al. Interrelationship between estimates of adiposity and body fat distribution with metabolic and hemostatic parameters in obese children. *Metabol Clin Exp* 2001; **50**(6):681–7.
58. McGill HC Jr, McMahan CA, Herderick EE et al. Obesity accelerates the progression of coronary atherosclerosis in young men. *Circulation* 2002; **105**(23):2712–18.
59. Pinhas-Hamiel O, Dolan LM, Daniels SR, Standiford D, Khoury PR, Zeitler P. Increased incidence of non-insulin-dependent diabetes mellitus among adolescents. *J Pediatr* 1996; **128**(5 Pt 1):608–15.
60. Pinhas-Hamiel O, Dolan LM, Zeitler PS. Diabetic ketoacidosis among obese African-American adolescents with NIDDM. *Diabetes Care* 1997; **20**(4):484–6.
61. Taha DR, Castells S, Umpaichitra V, Bastian W, Banerji MA. Beta-cell response to intravenous glucagon in African-American and Hispanic children with type 2 diabetes mellitus. *J Pediatr Endocrinol* 2002; **15**(1):59–67.
62. Marchesini G, Forlani G. NASH: from liver diseases to metabolic disorders and back to clinical hepatology. *Hepatology* 2002; **35**(2):497–9.
63. Ludwig J, Viggiano TR, McGill DB, Oh BJ. Nonalcoholic steatohepatitis: Mayo Clinic experiences with a hitherto unnamed disease. *Mayo Clin Proc* 1980; **55**(7):434–8.
64. Chitturi S, Abeygunasekera S, Farrell GC et al. NASH and insulin resistance: insulin hypersecretion and specific association with the insulin resistance syndrome. *Hepatology* 2002; **35**(2):373–9.
65. Marchesini G, Brizi M, Bianchi G et al. Nonalcoholic fatty liver disease: a feature of the metabolic syndrome. *Diabetes* 2001; **50**(8):1844–50.
66. Pagano G, Pacini G, Musso G et al. Nonalcoholic steatohepatitis, insulin resistance, and metabolic syndrome: further evidence for an etiologic association. *Hepatology* 2002; **35**(2):367–72.

67. de Marco R, Locatelli F, Zoppini G, Verlato G, Bonora E, Muggeo M. Cause-specific mortality in type 2 diabetes. The Verona Diabetes Study. *Diabetes Care* 1999; **22**(5):756–61.
68. Day CP, James OF. Steatohepatitis: a tale of two "hits"? *Gastroenterology* 1998; **114**(4):842–5.
69. Franzese A, Vajro P, Argenziano A *et al*. Liver involvement in obese children. Ultrasonography and liver enzyme levels at diagnosis and during follow-up in an Italian population. *Digest Dis Sci* 1997; **42**(7):1428–32.
70. Tazawa Y, Noguchi H, Nishinomiya F, Takada G. Serum alanine aminotransferase activity in obese children. *Acta Paediatrica* 1997; **86**(3):238–41.
71. Rashid M, Roberts EA. Nonalcoholic steatohepatitis in children. *J Pediatr Gastroenterol Nutr* 2000; **30**(1):48–53.
72. Lavine JE. Vitamin E treatment of nonalcoholic steatohepatitis in children: a pilot study. *J Pediatr* 2000; **136**(6):734–8.
73. Willi SM, McBurney P, Kennedy A, Wojciechowski B, Garvey WT. Ketosis-prone NIDDM in African-American children. *Diabetes* 1997; **47**(suppl 1):A67.
74. Winter WE, Nakamura M, House DV. Monogenic diabetes mellitus in youth. The MODY syndromes. *Endocrinol Metabol Clin N Am* 1999; **28**(4):765–85.
75. Banerji MA. Impaired beta-cell and alpha-cell function in African-American children with type 2 diabetes mellitus – "Flatbush diabetes". *J Pediatr Endocrinol* 2002; **15**(suppl 1):493–501.
76. Dean HJ, Mundy RL, Moffatt M. Non-insulin-dependent diabetes mellitus in Indian children in Manitoba. *Can Med Assoc* 1992; **147**:52–7.
77. Scott CR, Smith JM, Cradock MM, Pihoker C. Characteristics of youth-onset non-insulin dependent diabetes mellitus and insulin dependent diabetes mellitus at diagnosis. *Pediatrics* 1997; **100**:84–91.
78. Glaser NS, Jones KL. Non-insulin-dependent diabetes mellitus in Mexican-American Children. *West J Med* 1998; **168**:11–16.
79. Neufeld ND, Raffel LJ, Landon C, Chen YD, Vadheim CM. Early presentation of type 2 diabetes in Mexican-American youth. *Diabetes Care* 1998; **21**(1):80–6.
80. Onyemere K, Lipton R, Baumann E, Silverman B, Brodsky I. Onset features of insulin-treated atypical type 1 and early onset type 2 diabetes in African American and Latino children. *Diabetes* 1998; **47**(suppl 1):A25.
81. Zuhri-Yafi MI, Brosnan P, Hardin DS. Treatment of type 2 diabetes mellitus in children and adolescents. *J Pediatr Endocrinol Metabol* 2002; **15**(suppl 1):541–6.
82. Fajans SS, Bell GI, Polonsky KS. Molecular mechanisms and clinical pathophysiology of maturity-onset diabetes of the young. *N Engl J Med* 2001; **345**(13):971–80.
83. Hattersley AT. Diagnosis of maturity-onset diabetes of the young in the pediatric diabetes clinic. *J Pediatr Endocrinol* 2000; **13**(suppl 6):1411–17.
84. Sayeed MA, Hussain MZ, Banu A, Rumi MAK, Azad Khan AK. Prevalence of diabetes in a suburban population of Bangladesh. *Diabetes Res Clin* 1997; **34**:149–55.

chapter 9

Treatment of type 2 diabetes

Susan A Phillips and Kenneth L Jones

Introduction

Type 2 diabetes mellitus has moved from the status of a disease which rarely occurs in children, to one that is reaching epidemic proportions.[1,2] This change is requiring physicians who treat children to learn about the diagnosis, treatment, and prevention of this 'new disease'. It is now important to recognize not only the microvascular complications of insulin-deficient type 1 diabetes but also to address and prevent the macrovascular complications such as arteriosclerotic, cardiovascular, and peripheral vascular occlusive disorders associated with the insulin resistant syndrome (IRS) and type 2 diabetes. One must also consider the therapy of the other disorders frequently associated with these conditions, including hypertension, obesity, dyslipidemia, ovarian hyperandrogenemia, and nonalcoholic steatohepatititis (NASH). This discussion will deal only with the management of the hyperglycemia; therapy of co-morbid conditions will be mentioned only briefly, as it is beyond the scope of this chapter.

This chapter begins with the general therapeutic goals in children with type 2 diabetes, moving then to the specifics of glycemic management. When relevant, these approaches to glycemic management in type 2 diabetes will be compared and contrasted to those usually employed in treating type 1 diabetes. The methods to achieve glycemic control discussed here are presented in the light of the underlying pathophysiology of type 2 diabetes and include methods of and success of lifestyle changes.

We then move to a more extensive review of the use of oral antidiabetic drugs, their categorization, mechanisms of action, efficacy, and side effects. Monotherapy and combination therapy with the various agents are reviewed. Insulin therapy is discussed, with particular emphasis on the differences in insulin regimens from those traditionally employed in intensive therapy of type 1 diabetes.

A range of other topics are reviewed, including a number of clinical situations more frequently encountered in pediatric type 2 diabetes subjects: the treatment of the child who is acutely ill at diagnosis; treatment of patients in whom a certain diagnosis of type 1 or type 2 cannot be made; and the transition from insulin to oral agents in patients newly diagnosed with type 2 diabetes.

Because of the recent emergence of type 2 diabetes as a significant problem in children, there is a relative lack of data about its therapy in the young. As a result, we draw heavily on the extensive published experience with this disorder in adults. This experience, however, is often obtained in elderly adults, and may not always be directly applicable to children or, in view of the age differential, relevant to their therapy.

Differences from the type 1 model

Most pediatricians are familiar with the acute and chronic treatment of type 1 diabetes. They have, almost certainly, treated ketoacidosis and hypoglycemic reactions during their residencies and in their practices. Most also have experience with education of the child with new-onset type 1 diabetes and his or her family. The generally accepted goals of therapy are the prevention of diabetic ketoacidosis (DKA), avoidance of significant or frequent hypoglycemia, and the prevention of microvascular complications such as retinopathy, nephropathy, and neuropathy.

The Diabetes Control and Complications Trial (DCCT) established the importance of intensive therapy to accomplish tight glycemic control.[3] This study also confirmed that the success of this therapy could be followed and judged by measuring HbA_{1C} levels.[4] It has recently been reported that early, intensive control has a prolonged beneficial effect on delaying the development of microvascular complications.[5] With type 1 diabetes, an insulinopenic state, glycemic management is accomplished primarily with insulin replacement. Though they may vary in some details, most centers prescribe multiple daily insulin injections or continuous subcutaneous insulin infusion pumps. The treatment regimen also requires intensive and continuous education, frequent self-monitoring of blood glucose (SMBG), and carbohydrate counting. Insulin dose adjustments can then be made based on blood sugar, carbohydrate intake, and individual variation in insulin sensitivity.[6] The importance of frequent contact between the treatment center and patient and/or parent is well established.

Tight glycemic control is no less important in the therapy of type 2 diabetes,[7] though the methodology used differs in some respects. The primary metabolic defect of type 2 diabetes is insulin resistance in association with a relative and progressive deficiency in insulin secretion. This insulin resistance, present in many tissues, makes its primary contribution to hyperglycemia by reducing peripheral glucose uptake in muscle and failing to suppress hepatic glucose output. Additionally, resistance in adipose tissue to insulin-mediated suppression of lipolysis results in an elevation of free fatty acids (FFAs) and a further aggravation of hyperglycemia. The degree of insulin resistance observed in diabetic subjects may vary according to a subject's ethnic background, body mass index (BMI), and physical activity.[8,9] Pharmacologic intervention with either metformin, a biguanide, or a thiazolidinedione (TZD) has been successful in reducing insulin resistance in subjects with type 2 diabetes.[10]

Although information concerning the onset and progression of macrovascular disease is not yet available from individuals diagnosed in childhood with type 2 diabetes, the results of the DCCT have shown the considerable importance of microvascular disease progression in this population. Extrapolation of data from adults with type 2 diabetes suggests that the development of early macrovascular complications in childhood-onset type 2 diabetes is of concern. One recent follow-up study of type 2 diabetes in a young Canadian aboriginal population suggested that diabetic complications were devastating and occurred as early as the third decade of life (see also Chapter 4).[11] Though treatment of co-morbid conditions associated with type 2 diabetes is not discussed in this chapter, attention to the management of hypertension and dyslipidemia and their interaction with glycemic management are important topics for future investigation.

General goals of therapy

In the management of most forms of diabetes, there is a need to be concerned about the acute complications of hypoglycemia and keto-acidosis and/or development of acute hyperosmolar crises. Hypoglycemia, a major treatment concern in type 1 diabetes, is much less frequent with type 2 diabetes and is discussed later in association with specific thera-pies. Although DKA and hyperosmolar crises have been reported in chil-dren with type 2 diabetes,[12,13] they are uncommon, in our experience after initial presentation, but such crises have been reported.[14] About 10–15% of children and adolescents with type 2 diabetes present at diag-nosis with DKA, hyperosmolar crisis, or a combination of these states.[2]

The long-term goals in the management of type 2 diabetes are twofold: first, the prevention of microvascular complications, including retinopathy, nephropathy, and neuropathy; secondly, the prevention of macrovascular complications such as atherosclerosis of the coronary, cerebral, and large arteries of the lower extremities. These lead to myocardial infarction, stroke, and amputation,[15] and are the major causes of morbidity and mortality in adult subjects with type 2 diabetes. The development of these complications is multifactorial, but is influ-enced by associated hypertension, dyslipidemia, and hyperinsulinemia in addition to the effects of hyperglycemia.

Generalized approaches to therapy

The aim of therapy in type 2 diabetes is to specifically target the underly-ing metabolic defects of this disorder, which are obesity, abnormal insulin secretory function, and the insulin resistance present in the three primary insulin responsive tissues – skeletal muscle, fat, and liver. The sites of the metabolic lesions and the actions of the drugs used to correct them are shown in Figures 9.1a–c. The first approach is to reduce obesity through lifestyle interventions in diet and exercise. In addition, the introduction of an α-glucosidase inhibitor may be considered to delay carbohydrate digestion and absorption, reducing peak postprandial hyperglycemia. A second therapeutic approach is to address insulin secretory dysfunction with insulin secretagogues such as sulfonylureas or meglitinides. Alternatively, or if these secretagogues are ineffective, exogenous insulin can be initiated. A third approach is to address tissue-specific insulin resistance. Metformin can decrease hepatic glucose output and improve peripheral insulin sensitivity. Thiazolidinediones have been successful in improving peripheral insulin resistance in type 2 diabetes in adults; however, experience with these therapeutic agents is limited in children. These approaches are now discussed in more detail.

Specific approaches to the treatment of type 2 diabetes in children

Lifestyle changes

Lifestyle change has been the traditional first step in the therapy of type 2 diabetes in adults and has been extensively reviewed.[16] For this intervention to be successful, subjects must adhere to an intense program involving nutritional education, increased exercise, and a modified high fiber, low calorie, low saturated fat diet.[17,18] Although this approach may initially be successful in controlling hyperglycemia in adults, compliance is poor, weight loss is transient, and additional therapy is nearly always required. This 'need for additional therapy' implies that, for any form of therapy to be maximally effective, all patients with type 2 diabetes must incorporate at least some of the lifestyle changes outlined. One of the most encouraging pieces of information regarding the benefit of lifestyle change in type 2 diabetes comes from the recently completed Diabetes Prevention Trial.[19] This large study of a high-risk population of subjects with elevated fasting

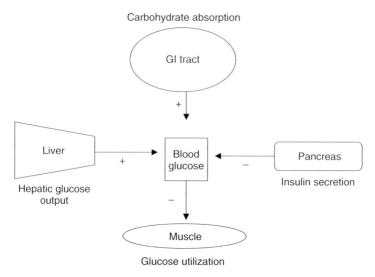

Figure 9.1a *Normal carbohydrate metabolism with glucose regulation accomplished by carbohydrate absorption in the gut; glucose utilization accomplished by normal insulin secretion and counterregulated by hepatic glucose utilization.*

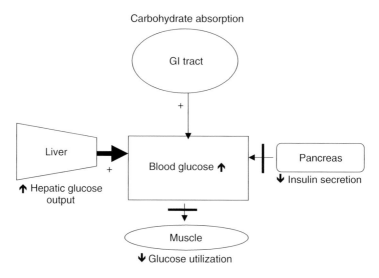

Figure 9.1b *Pathophysiology of type 2 diabetes. Insulin resistance decreases peripheral glucose utilization by muscle and fails to inhibit hepatic glucose output. Glucose utilization is further compromised by decreased insulin secretion by the pancreas. The result is increased blood glucose.*

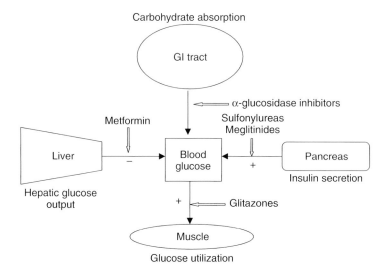

Figure 9.1c *Sites of action through which oral antidiabetic drugs lower hyperglycemia.*

and post-load glucose concentrations found that those randomized to lifestyle intervention had a 58% reduction in the incidence of diabetes compared with 31% for those receiving metformin.[19]

There is little information about the success or failure of change in lifestyle intervention in children,[20] and most of it is anecdotal. In general, the information suggests that, in primarily adolescent populations, lifestyle change has not established glycemic control. In a therapeutic trial of metformin versus placebo in children, described later, all patients were instructed in the principles of nutritional and exercise therapy, but only 7.5% of the placebo group maintained a level of glycemic control enabling them to complete the 16-week treatment arm without intervention. The remaining 92.5% required rescue with additional therapy to maintain the required degree of glycemic control.[21] Primary therapy with diet and exercise can work well under certain circumstances, such as in an institutional or structured home-care setting, and for developmentally delayed or impaired children. In these situations, caregivers can carefully control diet and activity programs.

Nutrition

Consultation with a dietitian familiar with children and with type 2 diabetes is important for all patients. The dietitian should assess the nutritional status and practices of the child and family and then counsel them to provide a meal plan which, at least initially, does not deviate in a major way from their usual eating practices. Changes made gradually, through subsequent appointments and interviews, frequently achieve compliance more successfully than does radical and rapid change.

Individuals providing counselling must be clear about the differences in the management of patients with type 1 and type 2 diabetes. Because obesity is a typical finding in type 2 diabetes and caloric restriction results in improved glycemic control and insulin sensitivity, modest caloric restriction and weight loss or maintenance are important goals: so is correction of the dyslipidemia, which frequently accompanies the metabolic syndrome or IRS. In general, calories from dietary fat should not exceed 30% of energy intake, and calories from saturated fat should not exceed 10%.[22] An effort is also made to limit cholesterol in the diet to <300 mg/day, and <200 mg/day if hypercholesterolemia is present.[22] Monounsaturated fats can be increased to up to 15–20% of total calories and may have beneficial effects on triglycerides and high-density lipoprotein (HDL). Protein should account for 15–20% of total calories, but may need to be adjusted for growth requirements. The remainder of calories is made up of carbohydrate.

Exercise

The beneficial effects of exercise on weight management, insulin sensitivity, blood pressure, serum lipids, and glycemic control, with or without the addition of pharmacologic agents, has been well documented.[17–19,23] As in adults, the key to success is finding an activity that each child likes and is willing to do. In this age group, there is also the potential to incorporate a school- or youth-based activity program. Cooperation and communication between schools and health care providers can encourage patients to participate more actively in scheduled physical education programs and can result in primary prevention.[24–26] Unfortunately, especially at this time of increasing obesity rates in young people, physical education programs in US public school systems are being reduced or made optional in many districts.

It is also helpful to encourage patients to increase activity at home through family walks and increased recreational activity. Often, however, the patients who are most likely to develop obesity and type 2 diabetes are from economically depressed populations with limited resources. These are also often single-parent households in which the lone parent does not have time to walk or exercise with the children. These children commonly live in neighborhoods unsafe for outdoor play and exercise. In many families, long hours viewing television or at the computer substitute for physical activities, further aggravating weight management.[27]

Oral antidiabetic drugs

As mentioned above and outlined in Figure 9.1, oral antidiabetic agents can function to improve insulin action in a number of ways: to increase insulin secretion, to suppress hepatic glucose output, to reduce peripheral insulin resistance, and to delay digestion and absorption of ingested carbohydrates. They will be discussed by category.

Insulin secretagogues (see Table 9.1)

Sulfonylureas

Comprehensive reviews of sulfonylurea (SU) treatment of adults discuss the pharmacology and mechanism of action of these drugs.[28,29] The cell surface receptor for SU has been cloned and shown to be linked to an ATP-sensitive K^+ channel in cell membranes which, when activated, triggers membrane depolarization, Ca^{2+} influx, and insulin secretion.[29]

In adults with type 2 diabetes, sulfonylurea therapy initially increases fasting and postprandial plasma insulin concentrations. The sulfonylureas, now in common usage, include first- and second-generation products, which act similarly but differ in potency and duration of action. All are bound to protein in the circulation, metabolized by the liver, and excreted in the bile or urine.

Candidates for therapy with SU must have residual beta-cell function. Approximately 20–25% of adults treated with SU show primary failure to respond. Of those who initially attain satisfactory glycemic control,

Table 9.1 Sulfonylureas and meglitinides

	Trade name	Recommended starting dose (mg)	Recommended maximum dose (mg)	Duration of action (h)
Sulfonylureas				
First generation				
Acetohexamide	Dymelor	125 bid	750 bid	10–14
Chlorpropamide	Diabinese	250 qd	500 qd	60
Tolazamide	Tolinase	100 qd	500 bid	12–24
Tolbutamide	Orinase	250 bid	1000 tid	6–12
Second generation				
Glimepiride	Amaryl	1–2 qd	8 qd	24
Glipizide	Glucotrol	5 qd	20 bid	12–24
Glipizide (extended release)	Glucotrol XL	5 qd	20 qd	24
Glyburide	DiaBeta, micronase	2.5–5 qd	10 bid	16–24
	Glynase Pres Tab	1.5–3 qd	6 bid	12–24
Meglitinides				
Nateglinide	Starlix	120 tid w/meals 60 tid w/meals if HbA$_{1c}$ near target		1–2
Repaglinide	Prandin	0.5 bid–qid w/meals	4 qid w/meals	1–4

bid = twice a day; tid = three times a day; qd = every day; qid = four times a day; w/ = with.

5–10% develop secondary failure with each subsequent year of treatment.[30] This failure may be patient-related, disease-related, or therapy-related. Patient-related failures include poor diet and/or medication compliance, and inadequate exercise. As type 2 diabetes progresses, beta-cell function declines, and disease-related drug failure ensues. Therapy-related failures result from inadequate dosage, desensitization, poor absorption, and/or antagonistic effects of other drugs.

Although hypoglycemia occurs less frequently in type 2 than type 1 diabetes, it is the major complication of sulfonylurea therapy.[31] Chlorpropamide and glyburide are more frequently associated with significant hypoglycemia than are shorter-acting preparations. Of the drugs that interact with sulfonylureas, most are not commonly used in children. One exception is trimethoprim, which may increase the risk for hypoglycemia by displacement of sulfonylureas from albumin-binding sites.[32]

The major toxicities of sulfonylureas involve the gastrointestinal system or skin. Up to 3% of users note nausea, abdominal discomfort, or vomiting and 0.5–1.5% develop rashes. Chlorpropamide is reported to be specifically associated with water retention and hyponatremia,[33] an effect that led to the use of chlorpropamide for treatment of central diabetes insipidus before the advent of synthetic vasopressin.

Meglitinides

Meglitinides, a new class of insulin secretagogues, were designed to lessen the risk of hypoglycemia by producing peak insulin responses that coincide with postprandial glucose excursions. Currently available meglitinides include repaglinide and the more recently approved nateglinide.[34] These drugs act by binding to the sulfonylurea receptor, inhibiting the ATP-dependent K^+ channel and causing a depolarization of the beta-cell, with subsequent secretion of insulin in the prandial phase. They have a shorter half-life, resulting in a quicker return to baseline insulin levels than is seen with sulfonylureas. With repaglinide, insulin concentrations return to baseline within 4–6 h[35] and, following nateglinide, within 2 h.[36] With this shorter half-life, there is a lower incidence of late postprandial hypoglycemia[37] than is seen with the more prolonged effect produced by SU.

Replaginide is taken shortly before meals in doses ranging from 0.5 to 4 mg. It is approved for monotherapy and for use in combination with metformin. Nateglinide is usually given in doses of 120 mg, 30 min before meals, as frequently as three times daily. For individuals who are close to, but not achieving their HbA_{1C} goal, a supplemental 60 mg dose of nateglinide may be given in combination with metformin.

As a class, meglitinides decrease the fasting glucose level by about 60 mg/dl (3.3 mmol/l) and the HbA_{1c} by 1.7–1.9%.[38,39] In individuals who are showing a poor response to meglitinide monotherapy, combination therapy with metformin has been proven safe and effective. In combination with metformin, repaglinide has induced an additional decrease of 1.4% in HbA_{1C}. Nateglinide plus metformin produces a decrease of 0.4% in individuals who have good control of their diabetes (HbA_{1C} <8%) and of 1.4% in those with a higher baseline HbA_{1C} (>9.5%).[40]

One disadvantage of the meglitinides is their frequent dosing requirement and resultant difficulty with compliance. Experience would suggest that this problem is greater in adolescents than in adults. Hypoglycemia resulting from hyperinsulinemia may occur, especially in individuals with low HbA_{1C} levels, but occurs less frequently than with SU.

α-Glucosidase inhibitors

One of the more difficult challenges in type 2 therapy is the reduction of post-meal hyperglycemia.[41] α-Glucosidase inhibitors act by competitively binding and inhibiting enzymes in the brush border of enterocytes that cleave oligosaccharides to monosaccharides, delaying the digestion of complex carbohydrates, and depressing the post-meal glucose peak.[42] Their role in diabetes management has been reviewed.[43] Because acarbose and voglibose are not absorbed, they have no significant systemic adverse effects, but do produce occasional abdominal pain, flatulence, and diarrhea, resulting from bacterial metabolism of oligosaccharides arriving undigested in the colon.[44] Miglitol is absorbed, but re-concentrated in the small intestine, so its effects are similar.

Studies in adults indicate that acarbose, as monotherapy, combined with diet can reduce HbA_{1C} by as much as 1.3%.[45] These drugs are not frequently used as primary or single drug regimens, but are employed as adjunctive therapy, usually in patients incompletely controlled by diet.[46]

Biguanides

Although discussed as a category, metformin is the only biguanide currently approved. Phenformin and butformin were removed from use because of their frequent association with lactic acidosis. Originally withdrawn from use in the United States with the other members of its class, metformin has been available in most of the developed world for nearly a half a century and was approved for use in this country again in 1995. Its primary action is to reduce hepatic glucose output, although it has a minor effect in reduction of peripheral insulin resistance.[47,48] Its safety and efficacy in type 2 diabetes in adults has been extensively reviewed,[49] and, in addition to its direct effect on reducing hyper-glycemia, it has also been noted to produce minor improvement in the diabetic dyslipidemic state and to enhance weight loss.[50,51]

Even before it had been subjected to a formal trial in children, metformin was the drug recommended for initial therapy of type 2 diabetes in this age group by an American Diabetes Association Expert Committee.[52] This recommendation was based on a general and positive experience of physicians who were using the drug 'off-label' in the 1990s.

A formal trial to ascertain metformin's safety and efficacy in children was initiated as a multicenter, randomized, double-blind, placebo-controlled program. In order to randomize the required 82 patients, it was necessary to involve 44 sites and to screen 481 subjects.[21] Nine of the sites were in Eastern Europe. Although it is difficult to know with certainty why recruiting was so problematic, strict exclusion criteria and the existing, prevalent, off-label use of metformin in diabetic children probably contributed. In support of the first point, 76% of the referred subjects were excluded because they fell outside the fasting plasma glucose limits of <126 or >240 mg/dl. Of the patients screened, 72% had HbA_{1C} values <7.0%. Only 11% of those referred were excluded because they were positive for one or more of the immune markers assessed (anti-GAD, ICA–512, insulin autoantibodies).

The demographic data from the enrolled group were very similar to those of patients described in earlier reports summarized by Fagot-Campagna *et al.*[2] In the study, approximately 70% of the metformin study patients were female, the mean age of the group was 13–14 years, fewer than 50% of all enrolled were white, and the mean BMI was high (approximately 34 kg/m²). The racial distribution was probably skewed from the usual US demographics of type 2 diabetes in children because 20 of the 82 enrolled patients were from European centers.

The study was designed to compare two groups of patients randomized into placebo and metformin groups. All patients received information about implementing lifestyle changes, which included advice about dietary modifications and increased, moderate exercise. Details of the study design and results are published.[21]

At the end of the double-blind treatment period, the mean fasting plasma glucose (FPG), adjusted for baseline, decreased by 42.9 mg/dl in the metformin group while increasing by 21.4 mg/dl in the placebo-treated patients. This improvement was confirmed by differences in the HbA$_{1C}$ at the end of the double-blind period. The mean values, adjusted for the baseline mean difference, were 8.6% in the placebo patients and 7.5% in those receiving metformin.

Patients receiving metformin experienced a mean 9.7 mg/dl decrease in serum cholesterol as contrasted with a 0.7 mg/dl increase in the patients receiving placebo. There was also slightly more weight loss and decrease in BMI in the metformin group, but none of these differences reached significance.

The study also established the safety of metformin in children. The number of patients experiencing at least one adverse event was higher in those receiving metformin than in controls (70% vs 60%), but the length of exposure to metformin was longer than that to placebo. As might have been predicted from experience in adults, the primary adverse events were in the gastrointestinal (GI) system. Nearly twice as many patients receiving metformin reported abdominal pain and nausea and/or vomiting as did those taking placebo.

The study confirmed that metformin was safe and effective for use in glycemic management of children with type 2 diabetes, and it has been approved by the FDA (Food and Drug Administration) for use in children.

Thiazolidinediones

This class of drugs acts to reduce peripheral insulin resistance, a key pathophysiologic feature of type 2 diabetes. The pharmacology and metabolic effects of these drugs have been extensively reviewed[53] and are not discussed here. Their actions and side effects are listed in Table 9.2.

Troglitazone was the first of these drugs to be employed in large clinical trials in adults with type 2 diabetes. The results were promising when it was used as monotherapy[54] or in combination with sulfonylurea[55] or insulin.[56] Fasting plasma glucose and HbA$_{1C}$ were reduced, as was insulin requirement. There were also potentially beneficial effects on lipid profiles, with increases in HDL cholesterol and decreases in triglycerides and free fatty acids.[57]

Unfortunately, the drug was found to have adverse effects on the liver, noted by increases in alanine transaminase, reversible jaundice,

---

Table 9.2 Thiazolidinediones: actions and side effects

Actions:
↑ Cellular responsiveness to insulin
↑ Insulin-dependent glucose disposal
↑ Hepatic sensitivity to insulin
↑ HDL cholesterol
Improves dysfunctional glucose homeostasis
↓ Blood glucose concentrations
↓ Plasma insulin levels
↓ HbA$_{1C}$ values
↓ Triglycerides
↓ Postprandial glucose and insulin levels

Side effects:
↑ Weight gain
↑ Cost
↑ Creatine phosphokinase levels
↑ Fluid retention
↑ LDL cholesterol
↑ Serum transaminase levels
↑ Fertility in women of childbearing age

and infrequent liver failure. Following additional evidence of associated liver failure, it was removed from use in March 2000.[58]

Other TZDs have now been approved by the FDA and are in general use. Trial results in adults with pioglitazone and rosiglitazone are published.[59,60] Clinical trials in children with both of these drugs are now in progress or being planned. In addition to their effects on blood glucose, rosiglitazone and pioglitazone have beneficial effects on dyslipidemia, blood pressure, and fibrinolysis.[61]

Rosiglitazone has a relatively short half-life of 4 h and is excreted primarily in the urine. As monotherapy, rosiglitazone has been very effective compared with placebo, reducing the FPG by 58 mg/dl at the lower dose of 4 mg/day and by an average of 76 mg/dl at 8 mg/day over a 26-week trial. At the higher dose, a reduction in HbA_{1C} of 1.5% was achieved over that in patients receiving placebo.[62] Rosiglitazone has been very effective when used in combination with SU and with metformin, reducing FPG and HbA_{1C} in patients who were stable, but not ideally controlled with maximal doses of either drug.[63,64] It can also be effectively employed in conjunction with insulin therapy, lowering both the FPG and insulin requirement.[65]

Pioglitazone, although different in some of its actions and in its metabolic processing by the body, has a similar therapeutic profile to rosiglitazone. While both of these drugs have been reported to have hepatotoxic effects, they do not occur with the frequency or severity seen with troglitazone.[66,67] Edema and reduction in hemoglobin have also been reported, as has weight gain. It is not known whether these effects are age-related, and whether they will be present, worse, or less significant in children. A detailed comparison of these agents is beyond the scope of this chapter, but the key features of their actions and side effects are listed in Table 9.2.

Insulin therapy

Insulin is an important and, ultimately, necessary agent in the therapy of type 2 diabetes. In adults, the natural course of type 2 diabetes begins with insulin resistance and evolves with the development of pancreatic beta-cell failure to an insulin-deficient state that requires the initiation of insulin therapy.[68,69] Although this 'late stage' may not occur during childhood, insulin therapy is still indicated in certain situations in this population. Insulin therapy is initiated at the time of presentation for acute metabolic decompensation and in cases of an unclear diagnosis of type 2 versus type 1 diabetes. Later insulin therapy is initiated for oral antidiabetic drug failure, poor compliance, and potentially for insulin deficiency developing with disease progression. It is also important to note that, as is the case with diet, insulin therapy in type 2 diabetes frequently differs from the regimens usually employed in type 1 diabetes. The types of insulin available for use and their approximate availability after injection are listed in Table 9.3.

Table 9.3 Types of insulin and their action

Type	Name	Onset	Peak	Duration
Very fast acting	Humalog Novalog	5–15 min	45–90 min	3–4 h
Fast acting	Humulin R Novolin R Velosulin Human	30–60 min	2–5 h	5–8 h
	Iletin II Regular (pork based)	30–120 min	3–4 h	4–6 h
Intermediate acting	Humulin L Humulin N Novolin L Novolin N	1–3 h	6–12 h	16–24 h
	Iletin II Lente Iletin II NPH	4–6 h	8–14 h	16–20 h
Long acting	Humulin U	4–6 h	18–28 h	28 h
Ultra-long acting	Lantus	1.1 h	No peak	Constant over 24 h
Mixtures (% NPH/ % regular)	Humulin 50/50 Humulin 70/30 Novolin 70/30 Humalog Mix 75/25	Varies	Varies	Varies

Situations requiring initial insulin therapy

Approximately 10–15% of children with type 2 diabetes are acutely ill at the time of diagnosis with DKA or with severe hyperosmolar states.[13,70] These patients must receive appropriate insulin and fluid resuscitation. Guidelines for therapy of DKA and hyperosmolar states are available and are not described here.[71] For children who are acutely ill with significant hyperglycemia, insulin should be started to quickly correct underlying metabolic derangements. 'Significant' may range from greater than 250 mg/dl to >400 mg/dl, depending on physician comfort. A transition period with continued insulin therapy is then recommended. This transition is important for stabilizing patients and, occasionally, for those physicians unfamiliar with this disorder, for providing the time to confirm the diagnosis of type 2 diabetes through documenting the absence of immune markers and the presence of ample C-peptide secretion. This transition period can be helpful in diagnosis, as the rapid decrease in insulin dose requirement characteristic of newly diagnosed type 2 patients is different from that seen in subjects with type 1 diabetes during the honeymoon period. Following establishment of a specific diagnosis, most patients can be transitioned to oral agents or a program of lifestyle change.

As has been suggested, often one sees patients in whom the differential diagnosis between type 1 diabetes and type 2 diabetes is not clear. It is also important to prescribe insulin for these individuals until a definitive diagnosis is made. With no specific test to confirm type 2 diabetes, there is a lack of universal agreement on how to establish the diagnosis or the criteria upon which the diagnosis is based. For clinical trials of drugs to treat type 2 diabetes in children, absence of immune markers and evidence of continued normal or increased insulin secretion are usually required as inclusion criteria.[21] In published reports describing the disease in children, however, patients are sometimes included as having type 2 diabetes although they are antibody positive.[72] In adult studies, patients originally classified with type 2 diabetes who were later found to be antibody positive are now frequently subdivided as having latent autoimmune diabetes of adults (LADA).[73,74] In the metformin study described above, among the children and adolescents with clinical diagnoses of type 2 diabetes referred for participation in a clinical trial, 10.8% were found to be positive for immune markers. In an expanded review of children referred for several studies of type 2 therapy, antibody-positive patients were slightly leaner and more likely to be Caucasian, but clinically resembled those enrolled in the studies who were antibody negative.[75] (See Chapter 2 for further discussion of these diagnostic issues.)

Insulin regimens for type 2 diabetes when lifestyle changes and/or
oral agents fail

Although the goals of insulin therapy are the same in type 1 diabetes and type 2 diabetes, the methods used may vary greatly. In the young patient with type 2 diabetes, endogenous insulin secretion is still present, so that supplementation may be all that is needed. Insulin may be used alone, or in combination with oral agents. Patients with type 2 diabetes are also less likely to experience hypoglycemia with insulin therapy. This subject has been extensively reviewed and is described only briefly here.[76]

Insulin supplementation   Most children diagnosed with type 2 diabetes have residual endogenous insulin secretion, but may benefit from basal insulin supplementation. These patients are usually mildly hyperglycemic and relatively easy to control. Before the availability of longer-acting insulin preparations, control was achieved by two or more injections per day of NPH. Now, longer-acting preparations, including human recombinant ultralente insulin and insulin glargine, are available and can provide single-dose basal coverage. In practice, however, most patients are treated with an oral antidiabetic agent rather than with basal insulin therapy.

Insulin in combination with oral agents   More commonly, insulin is added when glycemic control is not achieved on oral agents alone. Establishing a pattern of hyperglycemia can facilitate selection of an appropriate insulin regimen; this is frequently accomplished by having the patient SMBG. For example, with fasting hyperglycemia, a bedtime injection of NPH may be indicated. If the issue is primarily postprandial hyperglycemia, a short-acting insulin can be given as a pre-meal dose. Success can be monitored by SMBG.

Oral agent failure   A dependable indication for insulin therapy in adults with type 2 diabetes, once non-compliance has been excluded, is the loss of glycemic control, indicating beta-cell failure. In such patients, it is important to move to a more rigorous insulin routine of multiple daily injections or to the use of a continuous subcutaneous insulin infusion pump. These regimens, essentially responding to complete insulin deficiency, are similar to those used in individuals with type 1 diabetes, and they require similar attention to SMBG.

Insulin dependency occurs in adults with longstanding diabetes and, though well documented, is without an agreed upon etiology.[68,69] There is no reported, documented development of this condition in children, though certainly, with long duration of disease, it will occur in individuals with onset in childhood.

The frequent occurrence of oral agent failure often reflects failure to comply with the prescribed regimen. It is not unusual to resort to insulin therapy in adolescent patients with established type 2 diabetes, because glycemic control cannot be accomplished otherwise. Parents can participate in injection regimens, guaranteeing that the medication is taken, and achieving successful glycemic management. It is frequently more difficult to enforce an oral medication routine with the same success. It is also not uncommon that, with institution or reinstitution of injection therapy, a patient request is made for another trial of oral agents which then proves successful. Surprisingly, some adolescents prefer injections to oral medications.

With complete beta-cell failure, the insulin regimens usually employed are twice daily intermediate + short-acting insulin, given with breakfast and the evening meal. More intensive regimens use longer-acting insulins such as glargine[77] or ultralente[78] daily and short-acting insulins with meals. Ultralente can be mixed with short-acting insulins, but glargine must be given as a separate injection. These regimens are usually initiated with a 50/50 split of the two preparations and then adjusted based on blood glucose records.

Conclusions

In summary, childhood type 2 diabetes is reportedly reaching epidemic proportions as inactivity and obesity become more prevalent in children and adolescents. Physicians treating them must be aware of the diagnosis and the strategies necessary to prevent micro- and macrovascular complications. Although lifestyle interventions have been successful in adult type 2 diabetes and are recommended as first-line therapy in childhood type 2 diabetes, their efficacy remains to be proven in the latter population. An effective management plan usually includes lifestyle and pharmacologic interventions. The underlying pathophysiologic disturbances of type 2 diabetes – insulin resistance and relative insulin deficiency – provide the rationale for its treatment. Metformin, the drug currently most frequently employed in initial oral agent intervention, has been shown to be safe and effective for use in childhood type 2 diabetes. Other agents, including SU, α-glucosidase inhibitors, and insulin, have roles. The more recently introduced class of insulin sensitizers, TZDs, have been successful in adult type 2 diabetes, but their association with hepatic toxicity will require conservative use until trials proving safety and efficacy in children are completed.

The emergence of type 2 diabetes in the pediatric population, especially among minority populations, represents a daunting challenge to health care providers. If not prevented or adequately managed, the development of micro- and macrovascular disease in these children poses a significant public health concern for the future.

References

1. Rosenbloom AL, Joe JR, Young RS, Winter WE. Emerging epidemic of type 2 diabetes in youth. *Diabetes Care* 1999; **22**:345–54.
2. Fagot-Campagna A, Pettitt DJ, Engelgau MM *et al*. Type 2 diabetes among North American children and adolescents: an epidemiologic review and a public health perspective. *J Pediatr* 2000; **136**:664–72.
3. The effect of intensive treatment of diabetes on the development and progression of long-term complications in insulin-dependent diabetes mellitus. The Diabetes Control and Complications Trial Research Group. *N Engl J Med* 1993; **329**:977–86.
4. The relationship of glycemic exposure (HbA$_{1c}$) to the risk of development and progression of retinopathy in the diabetes control and complications trial. *Diabetes* 1995; **44**:968–83.

5. White NH, Cleary PA, Dahms W *et al*. Beneficial effects of intensive therapy of diabetes during adolescence: outcomes after the conclusion of the Diabetes Control and Complications Trial (DCCT). *J Pediatr* 2001; **139**:804–12.
6. Leahy JL. Intensive therapy in type 1 diabetes mellitus. New York: Marcel Decker, 2002.
7. Tight blood pressure control and risk of macrovascular and microvascular complications in type 2 diabetes: UKPDS 38. UK Prospective Diabetes Study Group. *BMJ* 1998; **317**:703–13.
8. Williams KV, Erbey JR, Becker D, Arslanian S, Orchard TJ. Can clinical factors estimate insulin resistance in type 1 diabetes? *Diabetes* 2000; **49**:626–32.
9. Arslanian S. Type 2 diabetes in children: clinical aspects and risk factors. *Horm Res* 2002; **57**(suppl 1):19–28.
10. Rosak C. The pathophysiologic basis of efficacy and clinical experience with the new oral antidiabetic agents. *J Diabetes Complications* 2002; **16**:123–32.
11. Dean H, Flett B. The natural history of type 2 diabetes diagnosed in childhood: long term followup in young adult years. *Diabetes* 2002; **51**:A24.
12. Dabelea D, Pettitt DJ, Jones KL, Arslanian SA. Type 2 diabetes mellitus in minority children and adolescents. An emerging problem. *Endocrinol Metab Clin N Am* 1999; **28**:709–29, viii.
13. Jones KL, Haghi M. Type 2 diabetes in children and adolescents: a primer. *The Endocrinologist* 2000; **10**:389–396.
14. Sellers EA, Dean HJ. Diabetic ketoacidosis: a complication of type 2 diabetes in Canadian aboriginal youth. *Diabetes Care* 2000; **23**:1202–4.
15. Nazimek-Siewniak B, Moczulski D, Grzeszczak W. Risk of macrovascular and microvascular complications in Type 2 diabetes. Results of longitudinal study design. *J Diabetes Complications* 2002; **16**:271–6.
16. Consensus Development Conference on Diet and Exercise in Non-Insulin-Dependent Diabetes Mellitus. National Institutes of Health. *Diabetes Care* 1987; **10**:639–44.
17. Hu FB, Manson JE, Stampfer MJ *et al*. Diet, lifestyle, and the risk of type 2 diabetes mellitus in women. *N Engl J Med* 2001; **345**:790–7.
18. Tuomilehto J, Lindstrom J, Eriksson JG *et al*. Prevention of type 2 diabetes mellitus by changes in lifestyle among subjects with impaired glucose tolerance. *N Engl J Med* 2001; **344**:1343–50.
19. Knowler WC, Barrett-Connor E, Fowler SE *et al*. Reduction in the incidence of type 2 diabetes with lifestyle intervention or metformin. *N Engl J Med* 2002; **346**:393–403.
20. Campbell K, Waters E, O'Meara S, Summerbell C. Interventions for preventing obesity in childhood. A systematic review. *Obes Rev* 2001; **2**:149–57.
21. Jones KL, Arslanian S, Peterokova VA, Park JS, Tomlinson MJ. Effect of metformin in pediatric patients with type 2 diabetes: a randomized controlled trial. *Diabetes Care* 2002; **25**:89–94.
22. Evidence-based nutrition principles and recommendations for the treatment and prevention of diabetes and related complications. *Diabetes Care* 2002; **25**:202–12.
23. LeMura LM, Maziekas MT. Factors that alter body fat, body mass, and fat-free mass in pediatric obesity. *Med Sci Sports Exerc* 2002; **34**:487–96.
24. Macaulay AC, Paradis G, Potvin L *et al*. The Kahnawake Schools Diabetes Prevention Project: intervention, evaluation, and baseline results of a diabetes

primary prevention program with a native community in Canada. *Prev Med* 1997; **26**:779–90.

25. Teufel NI, Ritenbaugh CK. Development of a primary prevention program: insight gained in the Zuni Diabetes Prevention Program. *Clin Pediatr (Phila)* 1998; **37**:131–41.

26. Gortmaker SL, Cheung LW, Peterson KE *et al.* Impact of a school-based inter-disciplinary intervention on diet and physical activity among urban primary school children: eat well and keep moving. *Arch Pediatr Adolesc Med* 1999; **153**:975–83.

27. Gortmaker SL, Must A, Sobol AM *et al.* Television viewing as a cause of increasing obesity among children in the United States, 1986–1990. *Arch Pediatr Adolesc Med* 1996; **150**:356–62.

28. Gerich JE. Oral hypoglycemic agents. *N Engl J Med* 1989; **321**:1231–45.

29. Ashcroft FM. Mechanisms of the glycaemic effects of sulfonylureas. *Horm Metab Res* 1996; **28**:456–63.

30. Gerich JE. Redefining the clinical management of type 2 diabetes: matching therapy to pathophysiology. *Eur J Clin Invest* 2002; **32**(suppl 3):46–53.

31. Heine RJ. Role of sulfonylureas in non-insulin-dependent diabetes mellitus: Part II – 'The cons'. *Horm Metab Res* 1996; **28**:522–6.

32. Ferner RE, Neil HA. Sulphonylureas and hypoglycaemia. *Br Med J (Clin Res Ed)* 1988; **296**:949–50.

33. Kadowaki T, Hagura R, Kajinuma H, Kuzuya N, Yoshida S. Chlorpropamide-induced hyponatremia: incidence and risk factors. *Diabetes Care* 1983; **6**:468–71.

34. Dornhorst A. Insulinotropic meglitinide analogues. *Lancet* 2001; **358**:1709–16.

35. Malaisse WJ. Mechanism of action of a new class of insulin secretagogues. *Exp Clin Endocrinol Diabetes* 1999; **107**(suppl 4):S140–3.

36. Hu S, Wang S, Fanelli B *et al.* Pancreatic beta-cell K(ATP) channel activity and membrane-binding studies with nateglinide: a comparison with sulfonylureas and repaglinide. *J Pharmacol Exp Ther* 2000; **293**:444–52.

37. Damsbo P, Clauson P, Marbury TC, Windfeld K. A double-blind randomized comparison of meal-related glycemic control by repaglinide and glyburide in well-controlled type 2 diabetic patients. *Diabetes Care* 1999; **22**:789–94.

38. Jovanovic L, Dailey G 3rd, Huang WC, Strange P, Goldstein BJ. Repaglinide in type 2 diabetes: a 24-week, fixed-dose efficacy and safety study. *J Clin Pharmacol* 2000; **40**:49–57.

39. Keilson L, Mather S, Walter YH, Subramanian S, McLeod JF. Synergistic effects of nateglinide and meal administration on insulin secretion in patients with type 2 diabetes mellitus. *J Clin Endocrinol Metab* 2000; **85**:1081–6.

40. Marre M, Van Gaal L, Usadel KH *et al.* Nateglinide improves glycaemic control when added to metformin monotherapy: results of a randomized trial with type 2 diabetes patients. *Diabetes Obes Metab* 2002; **4**:177–86.

41. Bastyr EJ 3rd, Stuart CA, Brodows RG *et al.* Therapy focused on lowering post-prandial glucose, not fasting glucose, may be superior for lowering HbA$_{1c}$. IOEZ Study Group. *Diabetes Care* 2000; **23**:1236–41.

42. Campbell LK, White JR, Campbell RK. Acarbose: its role in the treatment of diabetes mellitus. *Ann Pharmacother* 1996; **30**:1255–62.

43. Lebovitz HE. Alpha-glucosidase inhibitors. *Endocrinol Metab Clin N Am* 1997; **26**:539–51.

44. Hollander P. Safety profile of acarbose, an alpha-glucosidase inhibitor. *Drugs* 1992; **44** (suppl 3):47–53.
45. Hoffmann J, Spengler M. Efficacy of 24-week monotherapy with acarbose, metformin, or placebo in dietary-treated NIDDM patients: the Essen-II Study. *Am J Med* 1997; **103**:483–90.
46. Hara T, Nakamura J, Koh N *et al*. An importance of carbohydrate ingestion for the expression of the effect of alpha-glucosidase inhibitor in NIDDM. *Diabetes Care* 1996; **19**:642–7.
47. Bailey CJ. Biguanides and NIDDM. *Diabetes Care* 1992; **15**:755–72.
48. Fantus IG, Brosseau R. Mechanism of action of metformin: insulin receptor and postreceptor effects in vitro and in vivo. *J Clin Endocrinol Metab* 1986; **63**:898–905.
49. Bailey CJ, Turner RC. Metformin. *N Engl J Med* 1996; **334**:574–9.
50. Cusi K, Consoli A, DeFronzo RA. Metabolic effects of metformin on glucose and lactate metabolism in noninsulin-dependent diabetes mellitus. *J Clin Endocrinol Metab* 1996; **81**:4059–67.
51. Davidson MB, Peters AL. An overview of metformin in the treatment of type 2 diabetes mellitus. *Am J Med* 1997; **102**:99–110.
52. Type 2 diabetes in children and adolescents. American Diabetes Association. *Diabetes Care* 2000; **23**:381–9.
53. Saltiel AR, Olefsky JM. Thiazolidinediones in the treatment of insulin resistance and type II diabetes. *Diabetes* 1996; **45**:1661–9.
54. Fonseca VA, Valiquett TR, Huang SM, Ghazzi MN, Whitcomb RW. Troglitazone monotherapy improves glycemic control in patients with type 2 diabetes mellitus: a randomized, controlled study. The Troglitazone Study Group. *J Clin Endocrinol Metab* 1998; **83**:3169–76.
55. Horton ES, Whitehouse F, Ghazzi MN, Venable TC, Whitcomb RW. Troglitazone in combination with sulfonylurea restores glycemic control in patients with type 2 diabetes. The Troglitazone Study Group. *Diabetes Care* 1998; **21**:1462–9.
56. Schwartz S, Raskin P, Fonseca V, Graveline JF. Effect of troglitazone in insulin-treated patients with type II diabetes mellitus. Troglitazone and Exogenous Insulin Study Group. *N Engl J Med* 1998; **338**:861–6.
57. Fonseca V, Foyt HL, Shen K, Whitcomb R. Long-term effects of troglitazone: open-label extension studies in type 2 diabetic patients. *Diabetes Care* 2000; **23**:354–9.
58. Gitlin N, Julie NL, Spurr CL, Lim KN, Juarbe HM. Two cases of severe clinical and histologic hepatotoxicity associated with troglitazone. *Ann Intern Med* 1998; **129**:36–8.
59. Aronoff S, Rosenblatt S, Braithwaite S *et al*. Pioglitazone hydrochloride monotherapy improves glycemic control in the treatment of patients with type 2 diabetes: a 6-month randomized placebo-controlled dose–response study. The Pioglitazone 001 Study Group. *Diabetes Care* 2000; **23**:1605–11.
60. Lebovitz HE, Dole JF, Patwardhan R, Rappaport EB, Freed MI. Rosiglitazone monotherapy is effective in patients with type 2 diabetes. *J Clin Endocrinol Metab* 2001; **86**:280–8.
61. Parulkar AA, Pendergrass ML, Granda-Ayala R, Lee TR, Fonseca VA. Non-hypoglycemic effects of thiazolidinediones. *Ann Intern Med* 2001; **134**:61–71.

62. Patel J, Anderson RJ, Rappaport EB. Rosiglitazone monotherapy improves glycaemic control in patients with type 2 diabetes: a twelve-week, randomized, placebo-controlled study. *Diabetes Obes Metab* 1999; **1**:165–72.
63. Wolffenbuttel BH, Gomis R, Squatrito S, Jones NP, Patwardhan RN. Addition of low-dose rosiglitazone to sulphonylurea therapy improves glycaemic control in Type 2 diabetic patients. *Diabet Med* 2000; **17**:40–7.
64. Fonseca V, Rosenstock J, Patwardhan R, Salzman A. Effect of metformin and rosiglitazone combination therapy in patients with type 2 diabetes mellitus: a randomized controlled trial. *JAMA* 2000; **283**:1695–702.
65. Raskin P, Rendell M, Riddle MC *et al*. A randomized trial of rosiglitazone therapy in patients with inadequately controlled insulin-treated type 2 diabetes. *Diabetes Care* 2001; **24**:1226–32.
66. Lebovitz HE, Kreider M, Freed MI. Evaluation of liver function in type 2 diabetic patients during clinical trials: evidence that rosiglitazone does not cause hepatic dysfunction. *Diabetes Care* 2002; **25**:815–21.
67. Scheen AJ. Hepatotoxicity with thiazolidinediones: is it a class effect? *Drug Saf* 2001; **24**:873–88.
68. DeFronzo RA, Bonadonna RC, Ferrannini E. Pathogenesis of NIDDM. A balanced overview. *Diabetes Care* 1992; **15**:318–68.
69. Taylor SI. Deconstructing type 2 diabetes. *Cell* 1999; **97**:9–12.
70. Silverstein JH, Rosenbloom AL. Treatment of type 2 diabetes mellitus in children and adolescents. *J Pediatr Endocrinol Metab* 2000; **13** (suppl 6):1403–9.
71. White NH. Diabetic ketoacidosis in children. *Endocrinol Metab Clin N Am* 2000; **29**:657–82.
72. Hathout EH, Thomas W, El-Shahawy M, Nahab F, Mace JW. Diabetic autoimmune markers in children and adolescents with type 2 diabetes. *Pediatrics* 2001; **107**:E102.
73. Landin-Olsson M. Latent autoimmune diabetes in adults. *Ann NY Acad Sci* 2002; **958**:112–16.
74. Schernthaner G, Hink S, Kopp HP *et al*. Progress in the characterization of slowly progressive autoimmune diabetes in adult patients (LADA or type 1,5 diabetes). *Exp Clin Endocrinol Diabetes* 2001; **109**:S94–108.
75. Jones KL, Eisenbarth G, Klingensmith G, Fiedorek F. Comparison of type 1 marker positive and negative children with presumptive type 2 diabetes. Proceedings of the Endocrine Society's 84th Annual Meeting, 2002: P1–85.
76. Edelman SV, Henry RR. Non-insulin-dependent diabetes mellitus. *Curr Ther Endocrinol Metab* 1997; **6**:430–8.
77. Levien TL, Baker DE, White JR, Campbell RK. Insulin glargine: a new Basal insulin. *Ann Pharmacother* 2002; **36**:1019–27.
78. Campbell RK, White JR Jr. Insulin therapy in type 2 diabetes. *J Am Pharm Assoc (Wash)* 2002; **42**:602–11.

chapter 10

Long-term outcome of type 2 diabetes in adolescence

Yasuko Uchigata

Introduction

Type 2 diabetes mellitus has been reported in children in Japan, the United States, Pacific Islands, Hong Kong, Australia, and the United Kingdom.[1–6] Kitagawa *et al.*[2] reported that type 2 diabetes was more common than type 1 diabetes in Japan, accounting for 80% of childhood diabetes. The incidence almost doubled between 1976–80 and 1991–95.[2] The proportion of patients with early onset type 2 diabetes registered with the Diabetes Center, Tokyo Women's Medical University (TWMU) increased by 50% between 1960–1975 and 1986–1995 (TWMU database for 1960–1995).[7]

Thus, there is evidence that the incidence of type 2 diabetes mellitus is higher in young Japanese than in young Caucasians.[1,8] Since we first reported the young age of onset of many Japanese with type 2 diabetes attending our Diabetes Center in 1990,[1] it has become obvious that many develop severe diabetic vascular complications in their thirties[9] and show a higher incidence of diabetic nephropathy than that in Pima Indians with type 2 diabetes or Caucasian type 1 diabetes patients of comparable age.[10] Our findings on long-term diabetic complications of type 2 diabetes are felt to be representative of Japanese patients. Data on complications in other Asian and non-Asian populations with adolescent-onset type 2 diabetes are not available. In this chapter we describe the long-term outcome of type 2 diabetes in adolescence (early-onset type 2 diabetes) from our previous and later clinic-based observational longitudinal studies.

TWMU database

The TWMU database included all patients who had visited the Diabetes Center since 1960 and the Department of Pediatrics of the Tokyo Women's Medical University (TWMU) from 1960 to 1987. TWMU is located in the center of Tokyo. The TWMU differs from other hospitals and clinics in Japan in that it specializes in the consistent management of diabetic patients, with type 1 and type 2 diabetes mellitus,[11,12] from babies to old age, and takes care of diabetic patients daily in a multidisciplinary program of total care. The diabetes service includes the following divisions: care for children and adolescents; care in pregnancy; foot care; neuropathy care; nephropathy care with a dialysis unit; and an eye division for retinopathy. Before the mid-1970s, the greater part of the care was for children with type 1 diabetes. It was carried out by a pediatrician well versed in the management of type 1 diabetes in the Department of Pediatrics of the Tokyo Women's Medical University. From the mid-1970s, the TWMU started to take patients of all ages with diabetes. Approximately 500 patients visit the outpatient rooms of the Diabetes Center every day and 2700 new patients per year are usually registered at the Diabetes Center. One pediatrician and 20 internists have been authorized as diabetes specialists by the Japan Diabetes Society and 7 ophthalmologists take care of the outpatients at the TWMU. About 25,000 patients with type 2 diabetes and 1200 patients with type 1 diabetes were registered at the Diabetes Center between 1963 and the end of 1998. These numbers correspond to 0.4% of all Japanese type 2 patients and about 8% of all Japanese patients with type 1 diabetes.[13] Patients attending our center, which is a referral hospital, may be considered as representative of Japanese patients attending a diabetes specialized clinic.

In view of the large number of patients with type 1 and type 2 diabetes that developed at a young age, patients from TWMU represented a large proportion of the Japanese DERI (Diabetes Epidemiology Research International group) cohort.[14]

Diagnosis and classification of diabetes

The diagnosis of diabetes and the classification of diabetes type (type 1 and type 2) were made according to World Health Organization (WHO) criteria.[15] Briefly, type 1 diabetes was defined as the patient being prone to ketosis and requiring insulin therapy within 1 year after the diagnosis; type 2 diabetes was considered if the patient was found not to be ketosis prone, did not require insulin therapy for more than 1 year after the diagnosis, and/or exhibited preserved insulin secretion even when treated with insulin.

Among patients who first visited the Diabetes Center from 1970 to 1990 (n = 16,842), 1065 (6.3%) were identified as having early-onset type 2 diabetes who were diagnosed before the age of 30; this group served as a study population for the development of retinopathy (TWMU database 1970–90). Among patients who first visited the Diabetes Center from 1965 to 1990 (n = 17,236), 1638 (9.4%) patients with type 2 diabetes diagnosed before the age of 30 served as the study population for the development of nephropathy (TWMU database 1965–90). Type 2 diabetes was diagnosed because of symptoms (27%), other complaints (28%), or screening tests (45%). To confirm the diagnosis of the type of diabetes, serum C-peptide levels were measured in patients treated with insulin. As anti-GAD antibody, ICA, or IA-2 antibody measurements were not available in those days, they were not taken into consideration in the following studies.

Development of background and proliferative retinopathy

To study the development of background and proliferative retinopathy in Japanese patients with early-onset type 2 diabetes, 1065 Japanese patients with type 2 diabetes diagnosed before 30 years of age were recruited from the TWMU database 1970–90. Among a total of 527 patients who did not exhibit proteinuria or proliferative retinopathy at the first visit (baseline), 394 patients were recruited for the study, while 133 were excluded because they had not received continuous treatment.[16]

Table 10.1 shows the clinical and biochemical characteristics of the 394 patients at baseline. Age at diagnosis, gender, the duration of diabetes, therapy for diabetes, hemoglobin A_{1c} (HbA_{1c}), and proportion of smokers were similar for patients who participated and those who did not participate in the study.[16]

In this study, we used Fukuda's classification system, which is now the most commonly used classification system for diabetic retinopathy. Background retinopathy was defined as the presence of microaneurysms or dot hemorrhages (Fukuda A1, A2, and B1). Proliferative retinopathy was defined when patients had new vessels, vitreous hemorrhage, vitreo-retinal traction, or retinal detachment believed to be attributable to neo-vascularization (Fukuda A3, A4, A5, B2, B3, B4, and B5).

Predictors of background retinopathy

Of the 394 patients, 322 were free of retinopathy, and 72 had background retinopathy at baseline. The end point of the study was the development of background retinopathy[16] or the classification reached at the last examination. Of 322 who were free of retinopathy at baseline, 88 developed background retinopathy during a mean follow-up of 5.7 years.

Table 10.2 shows the predictive effect of independent variables on the development of background retinopathy. The known duration of diabetes, the baseline level and the mean levels of HbA_{1c} during the follow-up, and the serum concentrations of total cholesterol and triglyceride had significant predictive effects by univariate analysis (model A). The mean HbA_{1c} level had the strongest predictive effect for development of background retinopathy. Multivariate analysis (model B) revealed that only mean HbA_{1c} and duration of diabetes were significant independent predictors of developing background retinopathy.

Table 10.1 Baseline clinical and biochemical characteristics of the patients with early-onset type 2 diabetes who participated and those who did not participate in the study

Parameter	Subjects who participated	Subjects who did not participate
n	394	133
Percentage of men (95% CI)	54 (49–59)	57 (49–65)
Age at diagnosis of diabetes (years)	22.6 ± 5.6	23.6 ± 5.1
Age at baseline (years)	26.9 ± 8.2	27.7 ± 8.4
Known diabetes duration at baseline (years)	4.4 ± 6.0	4.1 ± 6.1
Percentage of patients with the following therapy for diabetes at baseline (95% CI):		
Diet alone	67 (62–71)	72 (64–80)
Tablets	16 (12–20)	14 (8–20)
Insulin	18 (14–21)	14 (8–20)
Hemoglobin A_{1c} (HbA_{1c}) at baseline (%)	8.5 ± 2.2	8.5 ± 2.6
Percentage of patients with background retinopathy (BDR) (95% CI)	18 (15–22)	9 (4–14)***
Percentage of current smokers (95% CI)	30 (26–35)	38 (30–46)
Body mass index (BMI) (kg/m^2)	23.0 ± 5.1	25.5 ± 5.6**
Percentage of patients with a family history of diabetes (95% CI)	61 (57–66)	54 (46–63)
Percentage of patients with a family history of vascular disease (95% CI)	12 (9–16)	16 (10–22)
Systolic blood pressure at baseline (mmHg)	116.4 ± 15.3	121.2 ± 15.6**
Diastolic blood pressure at baseline (mmHg)	73.1 ± 11.0	76.6 ± 12.3***
Total cholesterol at baseline (mg/dl)	195 ± 44	204 ± 43***
High-density lipoprotein (HDL) cholesterol at baseline (mg/dl)	51 ± 17	46 ± 12**
Triglyceride at baseline (mg/dl)^a	107 (69–182)	122 (75–189)***

Data are means ± SD, unless otherwise stated.
^{a} Data are median (interquartile range).
** $P < 0.01$ vs subjects who participated.
*** $P < 0.05$ vs subjects who participated.

Source: reference 16.

Table 10.2 Predictive effect of independent variables on development of background retinopathy (BDR) (cohort A)

Independent variable	P value	Hazard ratio[a]
Model A (univariate analysis)		
Age at diagnosis of diabetes	0.13	1.03 (0.99–1.07)
Age at baseline	0.0127	1.03 (1.01–1.06)
Duration of diabetes at baseline	0.0333	1.04 (1.00–1.08)
Body mass index (BMI)	0.82	1.01 (0.96–1.05)
Family history of diabetes	0.27	1.28 (0.83–1.98)
Family history of vascular diseases	0.74	1.11 (0.61–2.00)
Smoking	0.59	1.14 (0.72–1.80)
Mean HbA$_{1c}$	0.0001	1.25 (1.12–1.39)
Hemoglobin A$_{1c}$ (HbA$_{1c}$) at baseline	0.0464	1.12 (1.00–1.25)
Diastolic blood pressure	0.54	0.99 (0.97–1.01)
Systolic blood pressure	0.51	1.00 (0.98–1.01)
Total cholesterol	0.0397	1.00 (1.00–1.01)
Triglyceride	0.0214	1.00 (1.00–1.00)
Model B (multivariate analysis)		
Duration of diabetes at baseline	0.0027	1.06 (1.02–1.10)
Mean HbA$_{1c}$	0.00001	1.29 (1.15–1.44)

[a] Hazard ratio (95% CI) indicates alteration of risk per unit increase in independent variables shown in Table 10.1.

Source: reference 16.

The impact of mean HbA$_{1c}$ on the incidence of background retinopathy is shown in Figure 10.1 ($P<0.001$). The incidence increased remarkably when the mean HbA$_{1c}$ exceeded 8.5%. Comparison of the rate of retinopathy in our study with the Diabetes Control and Complications Research Group (DCCT) study was as follows: the incidence rate of background retinopathy at mean HbA$_{1c}$ level around 7% was 29.4 in our study (Figure 10.1) and 11.0 in the DCCT intensive-therapy group[17] and those around 9% were 71.3 (Figure 10.1) in our study and 40.1 in the DCCT conventional-therapy group.[17] The findings may suggest that Japanese early-onset type 2 diabetes patients are at high risk for diabetic retinopathy.

Incidence rate (per 1000 person-years)

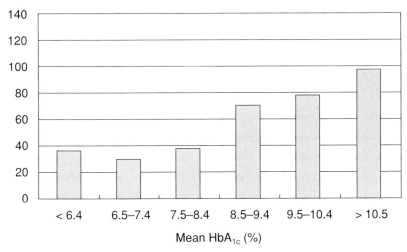

Mean HbA$_{1c}$ (%)

Figure 10.1 *Incidence rate for developing background retinopathy (BDR) in cohort A according to the stratification of the mean HbA$_{1c}$ level during the follow-up period. Incidence rate (per 1000 person-years) was calculated by dividing the number of patients who developed BDR by the observed person-years. Source: reference 16.*

Predictors of progression from background retinopathy to proliferative retinopathy

A total of 72 patients had background retinopathy at the baseline and 88 developed background retinopathy during a follow-up. Of the 160 patients with background retinopathy, 50 developed proliferative retinopathy. Table 10.3 shows the predictive effect of independent variables on progression. Only the mean HbA$_{1c}$ levels and the diastolic blood pressure level were significant independent predictors of progression from background retinopathy to proliferative retinopathy in multivariate analysis (model B).

The effect of mean HbA$_{1c}$ on the progression of retinopathy is shown in Figure 10.2 ($P<0.001$). The progression rate increased remarkably when the mean HbA$_{1c}$ exceeded 8.5%. When compared with the Diabetes Control and Complications Trial (DCCT),[17] the progression rates around HbA$_{1c}$ 7% were 27.8% in our study and 11.0% in the DCCT

Table 10.3 Predictive effect of independent variables on progression from background retinopathy (BDR) to proliferative retinopathy (PDR) (cohort B)

Independent variable	P value	Hazard ratio[a]
Model A (univariate analysis)		
Age at diagnosis of diabetes	0.35	0.98 (0.93–1.03)
Age at baseline	0.97	1.00 (0.97–1.03)
Duration of diabetes at baseline	0.53	1.01 (0.98–1.04)
Body mass index (BMI)	0.42	1.01 (0.97–1.09)
Family history of diabetes	0.46	1.25 (0.69–2.28)
Family history of vascular diseases	0.08	1.79 (0.93–3.44)
Smoking	0.49	1.22 (0.69–2.18)
Mean hemoglobin A_{1c} (HbA_{1c})	0.00001	1.42 (1.23–1.66)
HbA_{1c} at baseline	0.0237	1.21 (1.03–1.42)
Diastolic blood pressure	0.0169	1.03 (1.01–1.05)
Systolic blood pressure	0.089	1.01 (1.00–1.03)
Total cholesterol	0.50	1.00 (1.00–1.01)
Triglyceride	0.90	1.00 (1.00–1.00)
Model B (multivariate analysis)		
Diastolic blood pressure	0.0185	1.03 (1.00–1.05)
Mean HbA_{1c}	0.00001	1.43 (1.23–1.67)

[a] Hazard ratio (95% CI) indicates alteration of risk per unit increase in independent variables shown in Table 10.1.

Source: reference 16.

intensive-therapy group, and those around 9% were 69.5% in our study and 24.0% in the DCCT conventional-therapy group.[17]

The influence of diastolic pressure levels on the progression is shown in Figure 10.3. The highest tertile showed a two-fold higher rate of progression than the lowest tertile.

We found a slight elevation of blood pressure to have significant effect on the prediction of the progression from background retinopathy to proliferative retinopathy. Our finding may be comparable to the finding of the UK Prospective Diabetes Study (UKPDS) that tight blood

Incidence rate (per 1000 person-years)

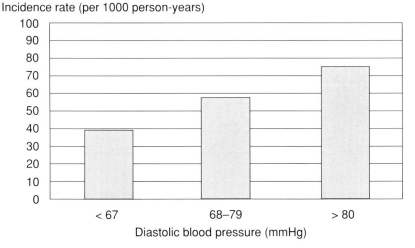

Diastolic blood pressure (mmHg)

Figure 10.2 *Incidence rate for progression from background retinopathy (BDR) to proliferative retinopathy (PDR) according to tertiles of diastolic blood pressure levels. Incidence rate (per 1000 person-years) was calculated by dividing the number of patients who progressed from BDR to PDR by the observed person-years. Source: reference 16.*

pressure control in older-onset type 2 diabetes patients achieves a reduction in the risk of progression of diabetic retinopathy.[18]

Comparison of the rate of retinopathy in our study with that of type 2 diabetes in other populations

No large-scale studies investigating the incidence of retinopathy in youth-onset type 2 diabetes have been reported. Of the small group of patients (n = 50) who developed type 2 diabetes between 1974 and 1997 before the age of 15 and were followed up at the Department of Pediatrics, Nihon University School of Medicine, 3 patients had proliferative retinopathy (duration: 27, 20, and 18 years) and 4 patients had macroalbuminuria or were on dialysis (duration: 27,20, 13, and 7 years).[19] When compared with old-onset type 2 diabetes, the progression rate from background retinopathy to proliferative retinopathy in this study was higher than for patients in the Wisconsin Epidemiologic Study of Diabetic Retinopathy,[20] Oklahoma Indian type 2 diabetes patients,[21] and Korean type 2 diabetes patients.[22]

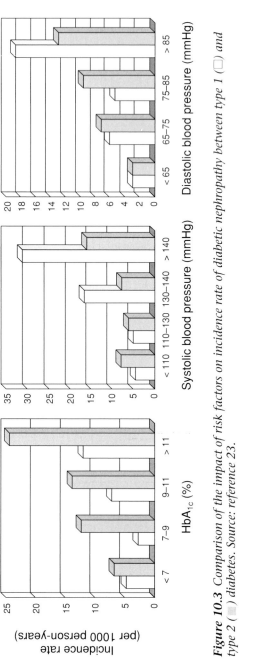

Figure 10.3 *Comparison of the impact of risk factors on incidence rate of diabetic nephropathy between type 1 (□) and type 2 (▪) diabetes. Source: reference 23.*

Development of nephropathy

The TWMU database 1960–90 was used to investigate the incidence of nephropathy in early-onset type 2 diabetes in Japanese patients[10] and the TWMU database 1965–90 was used to investigate the incidence of nephropathy in early-onset type 2 diabetes in Japanese patients and compared with those in early-onset type 1 diabetes.[23] Diabetic nephropathy here was diagnosed clinically when the following criteria were fulfilled: persistent proteinuria (protein in urine at the visit ≥300 mg/l); presence of retinopathy; and absence of clinical or laboratory evidence of disease other than diabetic nephropathy in the kidneys or renal tract. The end point of the study was the development of diabetic nephropathy or the status at the last examination.

Risk analysis for diabetic nephropathy

Table 10.4 shows the predictive effect of independent variables on the development of diabetic nephropathy.[23] The baseline level of HbA_{1c} and the systolic and diastolic blood pressures were significant predictive factors. The baseline HbA_{1c} level had the strongest predictive effect for development of diabetic nephropathy. The incidence of nephropathy increased with increasing HbA_{1c} levels and systolic and diastolic blood pressure levels (Figure 10.3).

The mean HbA_{1c} during the follow-up also had a strong predictive effect for development of diabetic nephropathy (Table 10.5) and the incidence increased with increasing mean HbA_{1c} level in a dose-dependent manner ($p < 0.0001$) (Figure 10.4).

Comparison of the incidence of diabetic nephropathy in type 2 diabetes with those in type 1 diabetes

Figure 10.3 also shows a comparison of the incidence of diabetic nephropathy in patients with either type of diabetes.[23] The incidence was higher in type 2 diabetes patients than in type 1 diabetes patients at every stratum of HbA_{1c} at the first visit. Only type 1 diabetes patients who had the highest blood pressure levels showed a significantly higher

Table 10.4 Clinical features of patients who did and did not develop nephropathy

	Developed nephropathy[a]	Did not develop nephropathy[a]	P values
Type 1			
Male (%) (95% CI)	30.1 (19.1–44.8)	39.3 (35.2–43.3)	NS
Age (years) at diagnosis of diabetes	15.3 ± 7.1	14.0 ± 7.5	NS
Hemoglobin A$_{1c}$ (HbA$_{1c}$) (%) at first visit	10.3 ± 2.0	9.4 ± 1.9	0.0002
Systolic blood pressure (mmHg) at first visit	122 ± 16	112 ± 11	0.003
Diastolic blood pressure (mmHg) at first visit	77 ± 10	70 ± 9	0.0001
Age (years) at diagnosis of nephropathy or at end point[b]	29.7 ± 7.2	29.2 ± 8.3	NS
Type 2			
Male (%) (95% CI)	55.2 (47.1–63.4)	55.3 (51.9–58.8)	NS
Age (years) at diagnosis of diabetes	23.1 ± 5.0	22.9 ± 5.3	NS
HbA$_{1c}$ (%) at first visit	9.6 ± 2.1	8.5 ± 2.2	<0.0001
Systolic blood pressure (mmHg) at first visit	122 ± 19	116 ± 16	0.04
Diastolic blood pressure (mmHg) at first visit	78 ± 11	74 ± 11	0.006
Age (years) at diagnosis of nephropathy or at end point[b]	36.2 ± 7.2	34.0 ± 9.9	NS

[a] Plus–minus values are mean ± SD.
[b] Definition of the end point is described in the method.

Table 10.5 Predictive effect of independent variables on the development of diabetic nephropathy in early-onset type 2 diabetes patients

Independent variable	P value	Hazard ratio[a]
Model A (univariate analysis)		
Gender (men vs women)	0.34	1.38 (0.71–2.66)
Age at diagnosis of diabetes	0.85	1.00 (0.95–1.06)
Age at baseline	0.15	1.03 (0.99–1.06)
Duration of diabetes at baseline	0.01	1.04 (1.01–1.07)
Insulin treatment at baseline	0.79	1.11 (0.51–2.40)
Body mass index (BMI)	0.003	1.08 (1.03–1.13)
Family history of diabetes	0.34	1.37 (0.71–2.66)
Smoking	0.67	1.15 (0.60–2.22)
Mean hemoglobin A_{1c} (HbA_{1c})	0.00001	1.56 (1.34–1.81)
Diastolic blood pressure	0.006	1.04 (1.01–1.06)
Systolic blood pressure	0.02	1.02 (1.00–1.04)
Hypertension	0.06	2.03 (0.97–4.27)
Total cholesterol	0.03	1.01 (1.00–1.01)
High-density lipoprotein (HDL) cholesterol	0.21	0.99 (0.97–1.01)
Log triglyceride	0.03	2.62 (1.09–6.31)
Model B (multivariate analysis)		
Mean HbA_{1c}	0.00001	1.63 (1.39–1.92)
Diastolic blood pressure	0.007	1.04 (1.01–1.07)
Duration of diabetes at baseline	0.04	1.04 (1.00–1.08)

[a] Hazard ratio (95% CI) indicates alteration of risk per unit increase in independent variables shown in Table 10.1.

incidence of nephropathy than early-onset type 2 diabetes patients with the same blood pressure ($p \leq 0.05$).

Figure 10.5 shows the cumulative incidence of diabetic nephropathy in 620 type 1 diabetes and 958 type 2 diabetes patients after post-pubertal duration of diabetes, according to the year of diagnosis.[23] The cumulative incidence was significantly lower in type 1 diabetes

Incidence rate (per 1000 person-years)

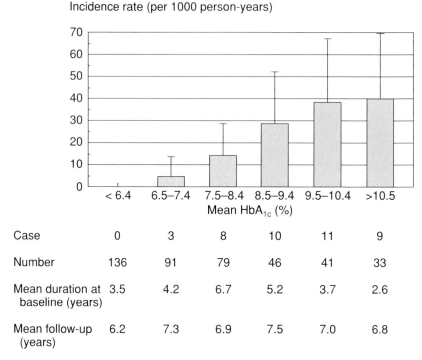

	< 6.4	6.5–7.4	7.5–8.4	8.5–9.4	9.5–10.4	>10.5
Case	0	3	8	10	11	9
Number	136	91	79	46	41	33
Mean duration at baseline (years)	3.5	4.2	6.7	5.2	3.7	2.6
Mean follow-up (years)	6.2	7.3	6.9	7.5	7.0	6.8

Figure 10.4 *Incidence rate for developing diabetic nephropathy according to the stratification of mean HbA$_{1c}$, levels during the follow-up period. Incidence rate (per 1000 person-years) was calculated by division of the number of patients who developed diabetic nephropathy by the observed person-years. Bars indicate 95% CI. Case indicates the number of patients who developed diabetic nephropathy. Number indicates the total number of patients in each range of mean HbA$_{1c}$ level. Source: reference 10.*

patients diagnosed in 1975–79 and in 1980–84, than in those with type 1 diabetes diagnosed in 1965–69, whereas it remained unchanged among type 2 diabetes patients when the various cohorts were compared. True duration of diabetes may be longer than the known duration in type 2 diabetes, but the difference between the true duration and the known duration is presumed to be less than a few years because type 2 diabetes rarely occurred before the age of 15 at that time. The rate of development of nephropathy for type 2 diabetes patients diagnosed in 1980–84 relative to type 1 diabetes

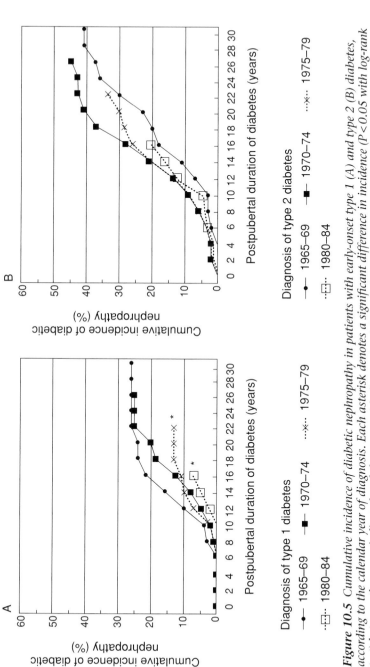

Figure 10.5 *Cumulative incidence of diabetic nephropathy in patients with early-onset type 1 (A) and type 2 (B) diabetes, according to the calendar year of diagnosis. Each asterisk denotes a significant difference in incidence (P<0.05 with log-rank test) between the group indicated and the group with diagnosis of diabetes between 1965 and 1969. Source: reference 23.*

patients diagnosed in the same period was 2.74 fold greater (95%CI, 1.17–6.41).

When the cumulative incidence of diabetic nephropathy was calculated after the first visit to the center, it was significantly higher ($p < 0.0001$) for type 2 diabetes than type 1 diabetes. This suggests that type 2 diabetes is the major cause of nephropathy in young-onset diabetes in Japan.

Existence of young-onset type 2 patients with severe diabetic complications

For several years, we have recognized that some young type 2 diabetes patients develop severe vascular complications rapidly. In most cases, we have found that these patients did not regularly visit a medical clinic until they suffered from visual disturbances or leg edema, at which point we identified the clinical characteristics of such type 2 diabetes patients.[9] The TWMU database 1970–90 was used for the analysis. A total of 1065 type 2 diabetes patients were divided into two subgroups: those who developed proliferative retinopathy before the age of 35 ($n = 135$) and those who did not ($n=930$). At the first visit, the 135 patients were not obese but had high HbA$_{1c}$ level and 75% of them had already been treated with insulin. Of these 135 patients, 53 (40%) were known to have type 2 diabetes before the age of 18.

Table 10.6 shows macrovascular and microvascular complications between the two subgroups.[12] The group who developed proliferative retinopathy before the age of 30 had subsequent progressive other complications: 60% developed diabetic nephropathy at a mean age of 31 years; 31% developed renal insufficiency at a mean age of 34 years; 23% underwent renal dialysis at a mean age of 35 years; and 24% became blind at a mean age of 32 years. Among the 31 patients who developed end-stage renal failure, 61% became blind and 29% developed atherosclerotic vascular disease at a mean age of 35 years.

It can be concluded that the subgroup with severe complications in their 30s was characterized by inadequate glycemic control.

Table 10.6 Microvascular and macrovascular complications in early-onset type 2 diabetes patients who developed proliferative retinopathy before 35 years of age and those who did not

	Group 1 (n = 135[13%])			Group 2 (n = 930 [87%])			P value
	n (%, 95% CI)	Age at diagnosis (years)[a]	Range (years)	n (%, 95% CI)	Age at diagnosis (years)[a]	Range (years)	
Proliferative retinopathy	135 (100)	29 ± 5	18–35	164 (18, 15–20)	45 ± 6	36–63	<0.0001
Diabetic nephropathy	81 (60, 52–68)	31 ± 5	19–44	70 (8, 6–9)	44 ± 7	27–61	<0.0001
Renal insufficiency	42 (31, 23–39)	34 ± 6	23–48	33 (4, 2–5)	46 ± 6	32–66	<0.0001
Renal failure requiring dialysis	31 (23, 16–30)	35 ± 4	26–41	19 (2, 1–3)	48 ± 4	43–56	<0.0001
Blindness	32 (24, 16–31)	32 ± 6	21–46	5 (0.5, 0.1–1.0)	46 ± 4	42–50	<0.0001
Atherosclerotic vascular disease	14 (10, 5–15)	36 ± 7	29–42	22 (2, 1–3)	44 ± 8	28–57	<0.0001

[a] Age at diagnosis is given as mean ± SD.

Source: reference 12.

Influence of urine glucose screening for schoolchildren and treatment interruption after diagnosis

As described above, it is obvious that inadequate glycemic control is the strongest risk factor for developing severe diabetic complications, which is caused by irregular visits to a medical clinic or interruption of treatment after the diagnosis.

A total of 283 patients were recruited; they were diagnosed with type 2 diabetes before the age of 18 and were registered in the Diabetes Center at TWMU from 1980 to 1998.[24] Among the 283 patients, 183 (64.7%) were diagnosed as type 2 diabetes by urine glucose screening for schoolchildren (school urine group). There were no differences of HbA$_{1c}$ level at the first visit, duration of diabetes at the first visit, the presence of treatment interruption, the history of initial hospitalization, and the presence of complications and the severity of them at the first visit between the school urine group and the non-school urine group (Table 10.7).

The patients were divided into two groups – the intermittent treatment group who had a history of treatment interruption (duration of interrupted treatment ≥1 year) and the continuous treatment group who did not have the history of treatment interruption. The former group had a significant higher increase of diabetic complications than the latter group (NcNemar method, $p < 0.0001$).[24] The school urine screening had no effect on protecting against diabetic complications and the treatment interruption was found to render the diabetic complications severe. These results show that treatment continuation is more important than screening or health checks to prevent diabetic complications.

Comparison of diabetic complications in patients with type 1 and type 2 diabetes

At the end of the 1980s we investigated the prevalence of diabetic retinopathy and nephropathy between two well-matched groups of

Table 10.7 Clinical characteristics of school checkup and other groups

	School checkup	Other	p
n	183	100	
Onset age (year)	14.8 ± 2.1	14.7 ± 1.9	0.6636
HbA$_{1c}$ (%) at the first visit	9.5 ± 2.8	9.4 ± 2.7	0.4079
Duration of diabetes (year)	8.5 ± 6.5	10.1 ± 7.6	0.2010
Intermittent treatment (−)/(+)	126/57	66/34	0.4752
Interval of intermittent treatment			
mean (year)	4.98 ± 3.27	5.79 ± 3.20	0.3260
Range (year)	1~15	1~15	
History of hospitalization (−)/(+)	95/88	55/45	0.6189
Complications (−)/(+)	128/55	63/37	0.2346
Score of complications			
Score 0	128	63	
1	19	7	
2	11	5	
3	4	4	0.0611
4	8	6	
5	6	3	
6	7	12	

Mean ± SD

Source: reference 24.

patients (average age at onset, 12 years; average duration before the first visit, 7.5 years) of type 1 diabetes ($n=42$) and type 2 diabetes ($n=97$), who developed diabetes before the age of 15 and visited us during 1980–1988.[25] The prevalence of simple and proliferative retinopathy was higher in type 1 diabetes than in type 2 diabetes. The prevalence of simple retinopathy in the type 1 diabetes group was higher than that in the type 2 diabetes group ($p<0.05$), while the prevalence of proliferative retinopathy in type 2 diabetes was higher than that in type 1 diabetes ($p<0.05$). The same investigation was performed using a cohort from the Department of Pediatrics, Nihon University School of Medicine.[26] This group also showed a higher prevalence of retinopathy in type 1 diabetes.

We are currently comparing the prevalence of the complications of those patients who developed diabetes before the age of 15 years and visited us between 1980 and 1998, with the late-1980s results described above, to examine the progress in the medical treatment of diabetes in the past two decades. The prevalence of simple retinopathy in type 1 diabetes was significantly lower between 1988 and 1998 ($p<0.005$), but there was no significant change in other complications (Figure 10.6).[27]

Prognosis of patients with young-onset type 2 diabetes

We are currently investigating the survival of young-onset type 2 diabetes patients. Okudaira *et al.* reported preliminary data on the survival status of 642 early-onset type 2 diabetes patients (by January 1, 2001) who were registered in TWMU from 1980 to 1990 and had visited for more than 1 year. The completeness of the follow-up for the survival status in the subjects was 74.0% (475/642) at the end of March, 2002.[28] Of 475 patients, 47 had died, as of January 1, 2001.[28] Main causes of death were cerebral vascular or cardiovascular diseases. Among Pima children aged 5–19 years who had normal or impaired glucose tolerance and type 2 diabetes, diabetic children also showed a high prevalence of cardiovascular risk factors,[29] which is expected to increase the number of cardiovascular diseases in young adults from high-risk populations.

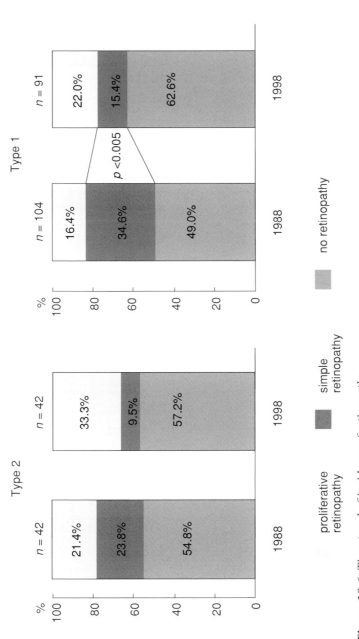

Figure 10.6 *Time trend of incidence of retinopathy.*

Conclusions

School urine screening was established under a rule of government in 1992 in Japan, although in some schools in Tokyo there had been a system to check urine glucose in addition to urine protein before 1992. The percentage of patients who were diagnosed as type 2 diabetes by school urine screening was increased from 1992; however, the frequency of the history of treatment interruption in the intermittent treatment group was similar to that in the continuous treatment group,[24] i.e., it is difficult to continue treatment of diabetes even in the patients who were diagnosed as type 2 diabetes at the initial stage of urine glucose detection only. It is clear that the patients in the intermittent treatment group have developed early onset severe diabetic complications.

It is suggested that it is impossible for all type 2 diabetes patients to continue treatment of diabetes. We have to think about other actions that patients should take so as not to develop type 2 diabetes and to protect/inhibit the development of diabetic complications. The simplest and easiest would be the promotion of lifestyle changes which encourage sports and exercise, thereby assisting adequate glycemic control. Japanese type 2 diabetes patients in adolescence are not as obese as their Caucasian counterparts; hence sports or outdoor leisure activities may be acceptable means of keeping adequate glycemic control.

Acknowledgments

The TWMU Database was begun by Dr Otani. Investigation of early-onset type 2 diabetes was then mainly performed by Drs Yokoyama and Okudaira, while investigation of the effect of intermittent treatment of diabetic complications was mainly begun by Dr T. Okada, who worked with us from April 1999 to March 2000 as a fellow from Department of Pediatrics, Kochi Medical School. I would like to thank all of my colleagues (Kasahara T, Otani T, Yokoyama H, Sato A, Muto K, Takada H, Okudaira M, Takaike H, and Osawa M) who have been involved in taking care of children and adolescents with diabetes in the Diabetes Center, TWMU. I would also like to thank Professors Yukimasa Hirata, Yasue Omori, and

Yasuhiko Iwamoto for their great support in their role as directors of the Diabetes Center, TWMU.

References

1. Otani T, Yokoyama H, Higami Y, Kasahara T, Uchigata Y, Hirata Y. Age of onset and type of Japanese younger diabetics in Tokyo. *Diab Res Clin Prac* 1990; 10:241–4.
2. Kitagawa T, Owada M, Uragami T, Yamauchi K. Increased incidence of non-insulin-dependent diabetes mellitus among Japanese school chidren with an increased intake of animal protein and fat. *Clin Pediatr* 1998; 37:111–15.
3. Rosenbloom A, Joe J, Young R, Winter W. Emerging epidemic of type 2 diabetes in youth. *Diabetes Care* 1999; 22:345–54.
4. Fagot-Gampagna A, Pettitt DJ, Engelgau MM *et al*. Type 2 diabetes among North American children and adolescents: an epidemiologic review and a public health perspective *J Pediatr* 2000; 136:664–72.
5. American Diabetes Association. Type 2 diabetes mellitus in children and adolescents. *Diabetes Care* 2000; 232:381–9.
6. Ehtisham S, Barrett T, Shaw N. Type 2 diabetes mellitus in UK children – an emerging problem. *Diabetes Med* 2000; 17:867–71.
7. Otani T, Yokoyama H, Sato A *et al*. Time-trend in the number of diabetes patients by age at onset and type of diabetes in Japanese patients diagnosed before the age of 30 [in Japanese]. *J Jap Diab Soc* 1999; 42:179–85.
8. Kuzuya T, Matsuda A. Family histories of diabetes among Japanese patients with type 1 (insulin-dependent) and type 2 (non-insulin-dependent) diabetes. *Diabetologia* 1982; 22:372–4.
9. Yokoyama H, Okudaira M, Otani T *et al*. Existence of early-onset NIDDM Japanese demonstrating severe diabetic complications. *Diabetes Care* 1997; 20:844–7.
10. Yokoyama H, Okudaira M, Otani T *et al*. High incidence of diabetic nephropathy in early-onset Japanese NIDDM patients. *Diabetes Care* 1998; 21:1080–5.
11. Yokoyama H, Uchigata Y, Otani T *et al*. Metabolic regulation and microangiopathy in a cohort of Japanese IDDM patients. *Diabetes Res Clin Prac* 1995; 29:203–9.
12. Yokoyama H, Okudaira M, Otani T *et al*. Existence of early-onset NIDDM Japanese demonstrating severe diabetic complications. *Diabetes Care* 1997; 20:844–7.
13. Akazawa Y. Epidemiology of Japanese patients with diabetes mellitus [in Japanese]. *J Jap Diab Soc* 1992; 50:7–13.
14. Uchigata Y, Asao K, Matsushima M *et al*. Comparison of mortality and end-stage renal disease (ERSD) between patients in one diabetes center and others in Japanese. *Diabetologia* 2000; 43:A256.
15. Harris MI. Classification and diagnostic criteria for diabetes mellitus and other categories of glucose intolerance. *Prim Care* 1988; 14:628–38.
16. Okudaira M, Yokoyama H, Otani T, Uchigata Y, Iwamoto Y. Slightly elevated blood pressure as well as poor metabolic control are risk factors for the

progression of retinopathy in early-onset Japanese type 2 diabetes. *J Diabetes Complications* 2000; **14**:281–7.

17. Diabetes Control and Complications Research Group. The effect of intensive treatment of diabetes on the development and progression of long-term complications in insulin-dependent diabetes mellitus. *N Engl J Med* 1993; **329**:977–87.

18. UK Prospective Diabetes Study Group. Tight blood pressure control and risk of macrovascular and microvascular complications in type 2 diabetes: UKPDS 38. *BMJ* 1998; **317**:703–13.

19. Owada M, Nitatori K, Uragami T. Characteristics and prognosis of type 2 diabetic patients diagnosed in childhood [in Japanese]. In: Oka Y, ed. *Toyoubyougaku*. Tokyo: Sindan-To-Tiryou Publishers, 2002: 53–63

20. Klein R, Klein BEK, Moss SE, Davis MD, DeMets DL. The Wisconsin Epidemiologic Study of Diabetic Retinopathy: X. Four-year incidence and progression of diabetic retinopathy when age at diagnosis is 30 years or more. *Arch Opthalmol* 1989; **107**:244–9.

21. Lee ET, Lee VS, Lu M, Russel D. Development of Indians in Oklahoma. *Diabetes* 1992; **41**:358–67.

22. Kim HK, Kim CH, Kim SW *et al*. Development and progression of diabetic retinopathy in Koreans with NIDDM. *Diabetes Care* 1998; **21**:134–8.

23. Yokoyama H, Okudaira M, Otani T *et al*. Higher incidence of diabetic nephropathy in type 2 than type 1 diabetes in early-onset diabetes in Japan. *Kidney Int* 2000; **58**:302–11.

24. Okada T, Okudaira M, Uchigata Y, Kurashige T, Iwamoto Y. Influence of urine glucose screening for school children and intermittent treatment on diabetic complications in early-onset type 2 diabetic patients [in Japanese]. *J Jap Diab Soc* 2000; **43**:131–7.

25. Otani T, Yokoyama H, Kanematsu S *et al*. Cross-sectional study of retinopathy in patients with non-insulin dependent diabetes diagnosed in childhood [in Japanese]. *J Japan Pediatr Soc* 1990; **94**(9):1973–7.

26. Takahashi H, Sato Y, Matsui M, Uragami T. Ocular fundus findings and systemic factors by type of childhood diabetes. *Nihon Ganka Kiyou* 1995; **46**(7):695–9.

27. Okudaira M, Uchigata Y, Otani T *et al*. The comparison of the diabetic complication in type 1 and type 2 diabetic patients diagnosed before the age of 15 who were registered in 80s with those in 90s. *J Pediatr Endocrinol* 2001; **13**(suppl 3):1040.

28. Okudaira M, Uchigata Y, Shimizu S *et al*. Investigation of prognosis of early-onset type 2 diabetic patients in Japan [in Japanese]. *J Jap Diab Soc* 2002; **45**:S95.

29. Fagot-Gampagna A, Knowler WC, Pettitt DJ. Type 2 diabetes in Pima Indian children: cardiovascular risk factors at diagnosis and 10 years later. *Diabetes* 1998; **47**:(suppl 2):A155.

chapter 11

The genetics of type 2 diabetes, MODY, and other syndromes

William E Winter

Introduction

The forms of non-insulin-dependent-non-autoimmune diabetes affecting children include:

1. type 2 diabetes
2. maturity-onset diabetes of the young (MODY)
3. mitochondrial diabetes and
4. other specific types of diabetes such as diabetes secondary to cystic fibrosis.

The genetics of each condition is discussed below.

Type 2 diabetes: genetic overview

There is convincing evidence that genetics plays a major role in the etiology of type 2 diabetes in adults.[1] Among people with type 2 diabetes, there is often a very strong family history of similarly affected individuals: familial aggregations of type 2 diabetes are common. Because lifestyle patterns that lead to obesity are so ingrained into everyday life and family habits, it is often difficult to separate nature versus nurture.

Concordance for type 2 diabetes between identical adult twins usually exceeds 90%.[2] This is much higher than concordance for type 1 diabetes between identical twins, which is 30–50%.[3] Dizygotic adult twins are concordant for type 2 diabetes in 3–37% of cases, illustrating a strong environmental contribution to the pathogenesis of type 2 diabetes.

Individuals with a sibling affected with type 2 diabetes display a relative risk for type 2 diabetes of 3–4. While this is not as high as the 10-fold relative risk for type 1 diabetes among siblings of type 1 diabetes probands, type 2 diabetes is much more prevalent in the general background population (approx 3 per 100) than type 1 diabetes (approx 1 per 300).

At a minimum, 25% of adults with type 2 diabetes have some form of family history of type 2 diabetes. As summarized by Rotter *et al.*[2], adult offspring of a parent with type 2 diabetes have a 4.0–9.7% risk for type 2 diabetes although this is likely to represent a very low estimate. Up to 76% will display an abnormal intravenous glucose tolerance test (IVGTT). Adults with a type 2 diabetes-affected sibling have a 2.4–11.7% risk for developing type 2 diabetes. Oral glucose tolerance tests in siblings of type 2 diabetes probands can be abnormal in up to 40% of cases. Children with type 2 diabetes commonly have affected parents.

As with other common diseases, the etiology of type 2 diabetes is multifactorial, involving both genetic and environmental factors.[4] Genetically, type 2 diabetes is also polygenic in that multiple genes, each with apparently only small to modest influences, combine to provide susceptibility to type 2 diabetes. Thus, type 2 diabetes is genetically heterogeneous. Conceptually, if the sum contribution of various hypothetical susceptibility gene alleles exceeds a certain threshold, type 2 diabetes can develop if the 'proper' environmental triggers are present, e.g., exogenous obesity and/or inactivity. The threshold for the development of type 2 diabetes is also dependent on the magnitude of the environmental trigger: more severe obesity probably lowers the threshold for type 2 diabetes and thus less genetic susceptibility would be required for the development of persistent hyperglycemia. The balance between genetics and environment in the genesis of type 2 diabetes also depends upon the number of susceptibility gene alleles carried in any individual as well as the magnitude of the environmental trigger(s).

Ethnicity has a major impact on susceptibility to type 2 diabetes. In the United States, type 2 diabetes is more common in ethnic minorities than in Caucasians. This is true in both children and adults: especially affected with type 2 diabetes are African-Americans, Hispanic-Americans, and Native Americans.[5–8] Fifty percent of adult Pima Indians in the south-western United States have type 2 diabetes, which is the highest diabetes frequency in the world.

Theoretically, type 2 diabetes might occur in children who have the strongest family histories of the disease and who are, therefore, genetically 'loaded' (e.g., predisposed) for type 2 diabetes who are also exceedingly obese and inactive, providing a high level of exposure to key environmental triggers. Type 2 diabetes occurring in the absence of obesity is more strongly familial than type 2 diabetes occurring coexistent with obesity.[9] Over the decades since World War II, children have become progressively heavier. This follows the national trend of rising obesity rates in adults.[10] One in four adults in the USA meets national criteria for the definition of the metabolic syndrome.[11]

Unfortunately no genetic studies directly address type 2 diabetes in children. However, because the pathophysiology is similar, the genetic etiologies may also be similar between children and adults who develop type 2 diabetes. Type 2 diabetes is believed to be expressed in children who may have stronger family histories of type 2 diabetes who also certainly achieve earlier and more profound levels of exogenous obesity and inactivity. Exogenous obesity is a consequence of the 'environment' (e.g., decreased exercise and increased caloric intake) and one's genetic susceptibility (e.g., the predominance, or lack thereof, of hypothetical futile cycles or the body's economy in maintaining the basal metabolic rate with a minimum of calories burned).

Type 2 diabetes: study designs

There are a variety of ways that the genetics of type 2 diabetes can be studied. Strategies for identifying type 2 diabetes-susceptibility genes are similar to those employed in other fields of genetics: population association studies, family linkage studies and affected sib-pair (ASP) analyses.[12] Population association studies determine if a particular gene allele (or alleles) occurs more or less frequently in a disease population than in an appropriately-matched control population. If the allele occurs more often in the disease population, the allele can be considered to be a susceptibility allele. If the allele occurs less often in the disease population, the allele can be considered to be a protective allele. Association studies are able to detect genes and their alleles that have major influences on the occurrence of a disease. Genes that have minor influences may not be detected with this approach.

Family linkage studies determine if a disease phenotype and a marker genotype or allele are co-inherited in a family. Large extended pedigrees of families with many affected individuals are required for such linkage studies. This approach assumes that a Mendelian dominant mode of inheritance is present. Other limitations include unavailability of family members for study (e.g., deceased relatives) and children who may not yet be affected but carry the disease allele.

ASP analysis establishes whether affected siblings within the same family share alleles at a particular locus more often than predicted by chance. It does not assume any specific manner of inheritance; however, large numbers of sib pairs are required for study and they must be clinically homogenous. Populations with higher rates of diabetes (and thus higher rates of affected sib pairs) may bias the genetic analysis because the genetics of random cases of type 2 diabetes will not be explored.

The genes examined for their potential relevance to type 2 diabetes (or other conditions) can include candidate genes or random gene markers in the form of a genome scan. The phenotypic expression of type 2 diabetes itself can be examined or the etiologies of type 2 diabetes can be studied, including: those factors that contribute to insulin resistance and those factors that contribute to insulinopenia.[13,14] Because the major force producing insulin resistance is obesity, the genetic study of type 2 diabetes, in part, can become the study of genetics of obesity. Indeed, genome scans for loci associated with obesity or body mass index (BMI) have been published.[14–22] Once the researcher entertains the manifest and central role of obesity in type 2 diabetes, the importance of the metabolic syndrome and its consequences begs our 'genetic' attention:

hyperinsulinism, hypertension, elevated plasminogen activator inhibitor-1 levels, dyslipidemia [hypertriglyceridemia, hypoalphalipoproteinemia, and dense low-density lipoprotein (LDL)], nonalcoholic steatohepatitis, acanthosis nigricans, hyperandrogenism, polycystic ovary syndrome, etc. Although mutations in leptin, the leptin receptor, prohormone convertase, pro-opiomelanocortin, and the melanocortin-4 receptor have caused monogenic forms of diabetes, these disorders are very rare causes of obesity in the general population.[23] Many fascinating candidate genes are under study in search of linkages to obesity or adiposity, including resistin,[24] peroxisome proliferator-activated receptor-gamma,[25] cocaine- and amphetamine-regulated transcript (CART),[26] beta$_3$-adrenergic receptor,[27] adiponectin,[28] hsp70-2,[29] uncoupling protein,[30] and islet 1 locus.[31]

Considering the complex metabolic functions of skeletal muscle, adipose tissue, hepatocytes, and beta cells, the minimal number of possible candidate genes is in the hundreds. Indeed, numerous studies have addressed the importance of various candidate genes in terms of type 2 diabetes, obesity, insulin sensitivity, and insulin secretion. Nevertheless, the candidate gene approach is limited by the investigators' preconception of which genes may actually be appropriate candidates. In fact, many susceptibility genes are unknown at the time of study [e.g., *CAPN10* in adult type 2 diabetes (see below) or transcription factor mutations in MODY]. A limited number of candidate gene studies in the field of diabetes have been successful (e.g., glucokinase and MODY2). Consequently, a more powerful way to address the genetics of any of the key variables [e.g., hyperglycemia (type 2 diabetes), obesity, insulin sensitivity, and insulin secretion] is necessary and is satisfied by the use of genome scans.[32]

Candidate gene studies in type 2 diabetes

Investigators have examined multiple candidate genes in population studies and in ASP analyses for their association or linkage with type 2 diabetes. There are several genes or loci where a positive association has been described with susceptibility to type 2 diabetes and there are no specific studies opposing that association. These genes/loci include the apolipoprotein A1, C3, A4 locus,[33] apolipoprotein B,[34] the beta$_2$

adrenergic receptor,[35] adiponectin,[36] chromosome 1 p36.3-p36.23,[37] chromosome 11 at D11S935,[38] hormone-sensitive lipase,[39] $K_{IR}6.2$,[40] lipid phosphatase SHIP2,[41] phosphoenolpyruvate carboxykinase,[42,43] PPARG[44] and prohormone convertase 2 (PC2).[45] There are more than 20 genes or loci that have been associated with type 2 diabetes in some studies but not in others. Many times these associations are population-specific: the association is identified in population 'A' but no association is detected when population 'B' is examined. Such 'controversial' type 2 diabetes-gene/loci associations are listed in Table 11.1.[46–81] In general, the strength of any of these associations is modest at best.

Table 11.1 Controversial genes or loci associated with susceptibility to type 2 diabetes

β_3-adrenergic receptor
Cholecystokinin type B receptor
Chromosome 1(D1S191)
Chromosome 12q [D12S321 and MODY3-linked non-MODY3 *(NIDDM2)*]
Chromosome 20q (D20S197, non-MODY1)
Glucagon receptor
Glucokinase
Glucose transporter-2
Glycogen synthase
Hepatocyte nuclear factor-1α
Hepatocyte nuclear factor-3β
Hepatocyte nuclear factor-4α
Insulin
Insulin receptor
Insulin promoter factor 1
Insulin receptor substrate-1
Islet associated polypeptide (amylin)
LIM/homeodomain (islet-1) ISL-1
NEUROD1
Ras associated with diabetes (RAD)
Skeletal muscle-specific glycogen-targeting subunit of protein phosphatase 1
Sulfonylurea receptor

Genome-scan studies in type 2 diabetes

Genome scans study the entire genome by examining markers placed at approximate 10 centimorgan (cM) intervals throughout the genome. To cover the human genome of ~3 × 10⁹ bp (10⁶ = ~1 cM; genome = 3000 cM), a minimum of 300 markers is required. The most useful markers are microsatellites. Such polymorphisms within populations are detected most readily by use of the polymerase chain reaction (PCR) with site-specific PCR primers flanking the microsatellite region. Automation of amplification and agarose gel separation of the PCR products has greatly aided this field in allowing rapid analyses of large populations studied at multiple loci.

NIDDM1: Calpain-10

The first pivotal genome scan to provide a novel and informative locus association with type 2 diabetes was performed in a Mexican-American type 2 diabetes population in Starr County, Texas.[82] In this county where 97% of the population is Mexican-American, the highest disease-specific diabetes mortality in the state of Texas was observed. Thirty-one percent of the gene pool was estimated to be Native American in origin. One hundred and seventy affected sibships including 330 diabetic siblings and 78 nondiabetic siblings were evaluated. The study employed 474 autosomal markers and 16 X-linked markers.

Evidence for linkage of type 2 diabetes with the microsatellite marker *D2S125* was discovered. *D2S125* was the most distal marker examined on the long arm of chromosome 2 (e.g., 2q). The maximum LOD score (MLS; LOD = likelihood of the odds) was 3.20, providing a *P* value of approx. 10⁻⁴. This chromosome 2 locus was named 'NIDDM1.' Proportionately approx. 30% of the familial clustering of type 2 diabetes was attributed to this linkage. This is similar in importance to the influence of the HLA locus on chromosome 6 (e.g., 40–50% magnitude of effect) in affording propensity to type 1 diabetes.

In examining non-Mexican-American populations, *D2S125* was not linked to type 2 diabetes in non-Hispanic whites or Japanese. In French subjects an ensuing investigation did not demonstrate linkage of *D2S125* (NIDDM1) with type 2 diabetes.[83] However, minimal evidence of linkage of *D2S140* with type 2 diabetes was reported [MLS: 1.196 (*P* = 0.016)]. Studies of Sardinians[84] and Finns[85] also failed to confirm linkage of type 2 diabetes to *D2S125*. Cox *et al.*[86] reported an interaction between *NIDDM1* and CYP19 on chromosome 15 with a weighted LOD score of 4.00 ($P = 2.1 \times 10^{-3}$) that provided susceptibility to type 2 diabetes.

In 2000, the gene responsible for *NIDDM1* was discovered.[87] The investigators performed positional cloning of chromosome 2q and *D2S125* by creating YAC, BAC, and P1-derived artificial chromosome (PAC) contigs. These centered on *D2S140* and spanned 1.7 megabases, which correlated with a 5.1-cM interval. In 10–20 unrelated type 2 diabetes-affected Mexican-Americans, ESTs (expressed sequence tags) and STSs (sequence tag site: detected polymorphisms) were recognized by DNA sequencing. Next, polymorphisms were tested for association with type 2 diabetes and for evidence of linkage.

Within the genomic interval containing *NIDDM1* there were seven known genes (GPC1, glypican 1; ATSV, axonal transporter of synaptic vesicles; AGXT, alanine-glyoxylate aminotransferase, liver-specific peroxi-somal; HDLBP, high-density lipoprotein-binding protein; NEDD5, neural precursor cell expressed, developmentally downregulated 5; PPP1R7, regulatory subunit of protein phosphatase 1; and S/T kinase-like) and 15 ESTs. Multiple polymorphisms of calpain-10 (gene name *CAPN10*) were discovered to be linked to type 2 diabetes in the Starr County population studied. At a common G→A nucleotide polymorphism (UCSNP43, University of Chicago single nucleotide polymorphism number 43) located in intron 3 of *CAPN10*, the G/G genotype was associated with type 2 diabetes. This study was a huge undertaking.[88]

Ubiquitously expressed in the fetus and adult, the family of calpain proteins functions as calcium-activated neutral proteases.[89] Calpain-like cysteine proteases operate as nonlysosomal cysteine proteases involved in processing, signaling, cellular proliferation, cellular differentiation, and insulin-induced down regulation of the insulin-receptor substrate-1 (IRS-1). Intracellular phosphorylation of IRS-1 plays a major role in the insulin-signaling pathway.

As mentioned above, calpain-10 is encoded by *CAPN10*, which spans 15 exons and 31 kilobases (kb). Two mRNAs are produced: 2.7 kb (the major mRNA product) and 4.0 kb (the minor RNA product). The composite cDNA sequence encodes 2620 nucleotides and 672 amino acids. Alternative splicing of the mRNA and translation leads to expression of proteins of various sizes: 672 amino acids, 544 amino acids, 517 amino acids, 513 amino acids, 444 amino acids, 274 amino acids, 139 amino acids, and 138 amino acids. The 672 amino acid protein is most abundant.

In addition to SNP-43, single nucleotide polymorphisms (SNPs) UCSNP 19 and 63 also affected proclivity to type 2 diabetes. Regarding the 43/19/63 SNPs, the greatest risk haplotype combination (112/121) delivered an odds ratio as high as 4.97 in Germans with lower positive odds ratios in Finns (2.55), and Mexican-Americans (2.8 in one group and 3.58 in another group). In Mexican-Americans and in Europeans the 112/121 genotype-attributable risks for type 2 diabetes were, respectively, 14% and 4%.

Concerning the epidemiology of type 2 diabetes, studies of calpain-10 were extended to many populations. A later study in Finns found no relationship between any *CAPN10* SNP (43, 56, 63) and type 2 diabetes.[90] In individuals and families of British/Irish ancestry,[91] SNP-43 was not associated with type 2 diabetes nor were the SNP-19 or SNP-63 polymorphisms. However, independently and when combined with the Mexican-American data, the C allele of SNP-44 was associated with type 2 diabetes. Samoans did not display an association between *CAPN10* SNPs 43, 19, or 63 and type 2 diabetes[92] nor did Oji-Cree First Nation's People of Northern Ontario[93] or Caucasians.[94]

In South Indians,[95] haplotypes based upon SNPs 44, 43, 19, and 63 revealed relative risks for type 2 diabetes as high as approx 6 fold; however, this 1112/1121 genotype is rare in that general population (only 0.9% of South Indians). Therefore in South Indians, *CAPN10* is unlikely to act as a major susceptibility gene for type 2 diabetes. To demonstrate a further lack of consensus in the literature, in the ARIC study reporting on middle-aged African-Americans, the *CAPN10* SNP-43 G/G genotype supported the Mexican-American data and was associated with type 2 diabetes,[96] whereas a study in Poles found that homozygosity for the SNP-43, SNP-19, SNP-63 haplotype 121 (121/121) was associated with type 2 diabetes.[97] In studies of another phenotype, *CAPN10* SNP-43 was not associated with extreme early-onset obesity.[98] There is preliminary data that natural selection at the *CAPN10* locus has occurred evolutionarily in Europeans and Asians but not in Africans.[99] These studies point out the challenges in attempting to map type 2 diabetes susceptibility loci.[100]

To examine the hypothesis that UCSNP-43 affected *CAPN10* mRNA expression, Baier *et al.* studied Pima Indians.[101] While there was no increased relative frequency of diabetes in Pimas homozygous for SNP-43 G (e.g., G/G), the nondiabetic genotypic G/G Pimas did display decreased rates of post-absorptive and insulin-stimulated glucose turnover that appeared to result from decreased rates of glucose oxidation. Furthermore, this correlated with decreased *CAPN10* mRNA expression in muscle in genotypic G/G Pimas. Thus, a pathophysiologic linkage was suggested between altered gene expression, altered mRNA expression, and decreased glucose removal from the body via decreased oxidation that could hypothetically produce hyperglycemia. A potential role for calpains in insulin secretion was demonstrated by Sreenan *et al.*[102] Mouse pancreatic islets treated with calpain inhibitors displayed increased glucose-stimulated insulin secretion.

In clinical studies of nondiabetic German adults typed as G/G vs G/A or A/A at SNP-43,[103] increased first-phase insulin response to intravenous glucose administration was recorded in G/G individuals as well as lower proinsulin to insulin ratios. This could suggest that the G allele is actually associated with better than normal insulin secretion. Alternatively, the G allele may be associated with insulin resistance and the higher first-phase insulin secretion is actually a compensatory beta-cell response to peripheral insulin resistance. In contrast with these findings, Hoffstedt *et al.* reported two-fold higher basal- and insulin-stimulated rates of glucose metabolism in adipocytes from nondiabetic SNP-43 G/G adults that predict increased insulin sensitivity in G/G individuals.[104] *CAPN10* SNP-43 appeared to modify adipose tissue β_3-adrenoreceptor function in obese individuals.[105] Elbein *et al.*[106] in studies of 63 Caucasian families with type 2 diabetes determined that SNP-19 and SNP-63 influenced fasting and post-glucose challenge insulin levels consistent with reduced tissue insulin responsiveness. British data also demonstrate an effect of SNP-43 on blood glucose levels and insulin secretory response.[107] There appears to be no doubt that one way or another calpain-10 does influence energy metabolism.

Calpain-10 may have metabolic and physiologic effects in addition to its proposed diabetogenic influences. An effect of *CAPN10* alleles on microvascular function was reported recently by Shore *et al.*[108] *CAPN10* may also influence cholesterol levels[109] and the development of polycystic ovary syndrome,[110] although this is controversial.[111]

In addition to calpain-10, various members of the calpain family appear to contribute to many diseases: in stroke and traumatic brain injury calpain 1 and 2 are overactivated; mutations in *CAPN-3* produce limb–girdle muscular dystrophy type 2A; and calpain 9 appears to function as a gastric cancer suppressor.[112] Lower levels of calpain 3 expression were reported to be associated with reduced carbohydrate oxidation and increased plasma glucose and insulin levels.[113]

NIDDM2

In a subsequent genome scan in western Finns,[114] a type-2-diabetes-linked region (termed '*NIDDM2*') was identified on the long arm of chromosome 12 (12q). Because this region of the genome includes the MODY3- gene hepatocyte nuclear factor-1α, Shaw *et al.*[115] were careful to determine if *NIDDM2* was MODY3 by examining the inheritance of type 2 diabetes in an Australian extended pedigree. Whereas the 12q region was linked to the inheritance of type 2 diabetes in the family studied, there were no mutations in the HNF-1α promoter region nor the 10 exons that were sequenced. Therefore *NIDDM2* can be described as a 'MODY3-linked, non-MODY3' type 2 diabetes susceptibility locus. In a study of early-onset autosomal dominant type 2 diabetes,[116] *NIDDM2* did not play an important role as a susceptibility locus. However, a locus 50 cM centromeric of *NIDDM2* was linked to type 2 diabetes. By studying 11 families with LOD scores of >1, this non-*NIDDM2* 12q susceptibility locus was narrowed to an interval between markers D12S1693 and D12S326.[117] However, there were no mutations of two genes within this interval, protein tyrosine phosphatase receptor type R and carboxypeptidase M. A subsequent study in the UK failed to genetically link chromosomes 12 or 20 with proclivity to type 2 diabetes.[50]

non-*NIDDM1-NIDDM2* genome scans

In addition to the studies described above, genome scans for type 2 diabetes susceptibility genes have been carried out in US Caucasians, Mexican-Americans, Pima Indians, Europeans, Ashkenazi Jews, and mixed populations.

A genome scan in US Caucasian Utahans was carried out by Elbein *et al.*[106] A LOD score of 4.3 was detected for a chromosome 1q21–23 locus near *APOA2* (the gene for apolipoprotein A2). In Mexican-Americans from the San Antonio Family Diabetes Study, a MLS of 2.88 was reported for a chromosome 10q microsatellite (D10S587).[118] This explained 64% of the variation in proclivity to type 2 diabetes. The MLS rose to 3.75 when adjusted for age-at-onset.

Etiologically associated with type 2 diabetes, fasting insulin levels in Mexican-Americans were influenced by a region of chromosome 3 (3p14.2–p14.1, LOD score = 3.07).[119] In Pima Indians, a chromosome 11q region was shown to influence the development of type 2 diabetes (LOD score 1.7) and BMI (LOD score = 3.6).[120] In nondiabetic Pima Indians, several loci were linked to glucose levels, insulin levels, and insulin action (Table 11.2).[121]

Genome scans in European populations have focused on Finns and the French. In FUSION I (the Finland–US investigation of non-insulin-dependent diabetes mellitus genetics study), chromosomes 20 (69.5 cM

Table 11.2 Mapping genetic loci that modulate metabolic parameters associated with type 2 diabetes in non-diabetic Pima Indians

Phenotype	Location	Microsatellite	LOD score
Fasting glucose	22q12–13	D22S270	1.75
Fasting insulin	3q21–24	D3S1764	1.48
Fasting insulin	4p15–q12	D4S2382	2.75
2-hour insulin[a]	9q21	D9S910	1.63
Insulin action	3q21–24	D3S1764	2.20

[a] During oral glucose tolerance test (OGTT).

from pter) and 11 loci displayed, respectively, MLS values of 2.15 and 1.75 for linkage to type 2 diabetes.[122] A chromosome 22 microsatellite (D22S423) was also significantly linked to type 2 diabetes (P = 0.00007). The chromosome 20 data were consistent with an earlier report from Ghosh *et al.*[123] FUSION II involved genetic analyses of a variety of metabolic parameters.[124] Body mass index was linked to chromosome 3 (MLS = 3.43), whereas insulin resistance was linked to chromosome 17 (MLS = 3.61). In the French study, diabetes or glucose intolerance demonstrated linkage to D3S1580 on chromosome 3 with an MLS of 4.67.[125] In this study type 2 diabetes in lean French subjects was linked to chromosome 1q21–q24 (MLS = 3.04).

The results of the genome scan performed by the GENNID (Genetics of NIDDM) study group were published in 2000.[126] Four population groups were examined: whites, Mexican-Americans, blacks, and Japanese Americans. Linkages to diabetes or impaired glucose tolerance were reported for chromosomes 3, 5, 10, 12, and X (Table 11.3).

Genome-scan analysis of Israeli Ashkenazi Jewish pedigrees demonstrated nominal evidence for linkage of type 2 diabetes to five loci on four chromosomes (4q, 8q, 14q, and 20q).[127] This paper supports the proposal that a locus on chromosome 20q does influence diabetogenesis. A genome scan of the Framingham Offspring Study using analysis of quantitative trait loci found two regions that influence glucose levels: one locus on chromosome 1p and one locus on chromosome 10q.[128] A

Table 11.3 Mapping genetic loci linked with type 2 diabetes or glucose intolerance in the GENNID study

Population	Chromosome	Microsatellite	MLS score
Whites	5	D5S140	2.80
	12	D12S853	2.81
	X	GATA172D05	2.99
Mexican-Americans	3	D3S2432	3.91
Blacks	10	D10S1412	2.39

genome scan in Japanese ASPs suggested novel type 2 diabetes susceptibility loci at chromosomes 7p22–p21 and 11p13–p12.[129]

In summary, there is no shortage of genomic intervals that may influence susceptibility to type 2 diabetes. Regions on chromosomes 1, 2, 3, 4, 5, 7, 8, 11, 12, 14, 20, 22, and X (Table 11.4) have been implicated in various populations.[130] This emphasizes the polygenic nature of susceptibility to type 2 diabetes where multiple genes, each with small to modest effects, influence the development of type 2 diabetes. It is likely that in each studied population, to different degrees different genes influence the development of type 2 diabetes. No single gene appears to exhibit a strong influence on the development of type 2 diabetes across populations.

Table 11.4 Overview of genome scans for linkage of type 2 diabetes

Year of the report	Population studied	Linked chromosome/ locus	Comments
1996	Mexican-Americans	Chr. 2:	*NIDDM1*, calpain-10 (*CAPN10*)
1996	Western Finns	Chr.12	*NIDDM2*
1998	Pimas	Chr. 11q	
1999	Utahans	Chr. 1q21–23	
1999	Mexican-Americans	Chr.10q (D10S587)	
2000	Finns	Chr. 11, 20, and 22	FUSION I
2000	Whites	D5S140 D12S853 X chromosome	GENNID
	Mexican-Americans	D3S2432	
	African-Americans	D10S142	
2000	French (lean diabetes)	D3S1589 1q21–q24	
2001	Ashkenazi Jewish	4q, 8q, 14q, and 20q	
2002	North American Europeans	1p, 10p	Framingham, USA

Maturity-onset diabetes of youth (MODY)

Genetically, MODY is defined as an autosomal dominant form of non-insulin requiring-nonketotic diabetes with onset before age 25.[131,132] Some definitions of MODY include the presence of measurable C-peptide or a duration of up to 5 years for non-insulin treatment following diagnosis. Using the 1997 ADA classification scheme, because MODY is an insulinopenic form of diabetes where specific molecular mutations have been identified, MODY is classified as a form of 'other specific types of diabetes: genetic defects of beta-cell function'. As opposed to type 2 diabetes, which results from insulin resistance and relative insulinopenia, MODY patients exhibit insulinopenia, although the degree of insulinopenia is not as severe as that observed in type 1 diabetes where, with established disease, C-peptide is not usually measurable.

MODY is predominantly a disorder of Caucasians and accounts for 1–2% of cases of diabetes in the United Kingdom. In the German district of Hesse, MODY cases represented 2.1% of cases of non-insulin-dependent diabetes mellitus (NIDDM). MODY may be most common in France, where 10% of white families with NIDDM express the MODY phenotype. MODY should be included in the differential diagnosis of 'mild' or incidental hyperglycemia.

A clinical MODY-variant termed 'atypical diabetes mellitus' (ADM) occurs in African-Americans.[133] Like classic MODY patients, ADM patients exhibit youth-onset diabetes (≤40 years old) that is inherited in an autosomal dominant pattern. However, ADM differs from Caucasian MODY because ADM presents acutely and requires insulin treatment for management of hyperglycemia and ketosis or even frank diabetic ketoacidosis. After months to years, ADM does remit to a non-insulin dependent form of diabetes. Unless the family history is patently obvious, it may be a challenge for the clinician to differentiate ADM from type 1 diabetes at disease onset.

Six genes have been linked to MODY in various families (Table 11.5). Five of the six genes are transcription factors: hepatocyte nuclear factor-4α (HNF-4α, MODY1); hepatocyte nuclear factor-1α (HNF-1α, MODY3); insulin promoter factor-1 (IPF-1, MODY4); hepatocyte nuclear factor-1β

Table 11.5 Classification of the MODY syndromes

Classification	Defect	Abbreviation	Severity	Frequency[a]
MODY1	Hepatocyte nuclear factor-4α	HNF-4α	+++	Uncommon
MODY2	Glucokinase	GCK	+	Common
MODY3	Hepatocyte nuclear factor-1α	HNF-1α	+++	Common
MODY4	Insulin promoter factor-1	IPF-1	++	Rare
MODY5	Hepatocyte nuclear factor-1β	HNF-1β	+++	Rare
MODY6	NeuroD1/Beta2	NeuroD1	+++	Rare

[a] As a cause of MODY.

(HNF-1β, MODY5); and neurod1/beta2 (NeuroD1, MODY6).[134,135] Hypothetically because transcription factors regulate gene expression, loss-of-function mutations in transcription factors impair insulin production, leading to insulinopenia of various degrees. Transcription factors also regulate pancreatic, islet, and beta-cell development.[136] Certainly, none of the MODY syndromes demonstrate the degree of severe insulinopenia that is observed in long-term type 1 diabetes.

The clinical penetrance of MODY in individuals with the transcription factor mutations is approx. 80% by age 40. Because many transcription factors are expressed in the liver, liver dysfunction might contribute to diabetes in MODY subjects. Transcription factors often operate in hierarchies where one transcription factor controls the expression of another transcription factor.[137] This appears to be the case concerning transcription factors that cause MODY. MODY2 results from loss-of-function mutations in glucokinase which is the major liver and beta-cell hexokinase.

MODY 2 and MODY 3 represent approx. 80% of MODY cases. MODY1 is uncommon and MODY4, MODY5, and MODY6 are rare causes of MODY. In terms of severity, MODY2 is the least severe form.[138,139] MODY4 is intermediate in severity and MODY1, MODY3, MODY5, and MODY6 are the most severe forms of MODY.[140] When diabetes in a family displays all of the clinical features of MODY but none of the described loci are linked to MODY in the family, 'MODY-X' is said to be present.

MODY1: hepatocyte nuclear factor-4α

MODY1 (HNF-4α, chromosome 20q12–q13.1) was initially described in the large RW pedigree.[141] MODY1 was the first transcription factor mutation discovered to cause MODY.[142] HNF-4α is normally expressed in the liver, kidney, intestine, and islets and serves as a key regulator of hepatic gene expression.

MODY1 displays insulinopenia[143] that is progressive with increasing age. MODY1 patients may eventually require insulin replacement although many of them are managed adequately for decades using oral sulfonyl-ureas. In MODY1 subjects, insulin secretion is not enhanced by glucose priming.[144] The fasting plasma glucose can be in the normal range; however, after glucose challenge, hyperglycemia definitely occurs. Insulin and glucagon responses to arginine are deficient.[145] Both microvascular and macrovascular complications occur in MODY1 patients. Approximately 10 HNF-4α mutations have been described.[146–148] HNF-4α mutations are rare causes of type 2 diabetes.[64,149] One estimate asserted that <0.0001% of adult type 2 diabetes cases resulted from HNF-4α mutations.[150]

MODY2: glucokinase

MODY2, resulting from glucokinase mutations (chromosome 7p15–p13), is the most common form of MODY in France (approx. 50% of MODY cases).[151] MODY2 is also a common etiology of MODY in Italy, being responsible for 58% of Italian MODY pedigrees. Glucokinase was the first molecular cause of MODY discovered.[152,153] Glucokinase functions as the glucose sensor of the beta cell and plays a role in hepatocyte glucose clearance.[154] MODY2 subjects exhibit a nonprogressive insulinopenia of prenatal onset with a reduction in birth weight of approx. 500 g compared to their unaffected siblings.[155] There is an approx. 60% reduction in insulin secretion and rightward shift in the insulin–glucose response curve.[156] Insulin response to arginine infusion is usually normal or near normal. There is an improved insulin response after glucose priming. MODY2 diabetes is relatively mild but does exhibit mild fasting hyperglycemia. Because of the mild nature of MODY2 diabetes, there is an apparent low rate of complications. There is an approx. 50% rate of penetrance of MODY2 by age 40. More cases are found when oral glucose tolerance tests (OGTTs) are carried out on family members.

More than 130 glucokinase mutations have been described.[157] Homozygous glucokinase mutations are very serious and cause neonatal diabetes.[158] This has been reported in one Norwegian and one Italian family. It is controversial to what degree MODY2 causes gestational diabetes mellitus.[159–161] Some studies have found that 3–6% of women with gestational diabetes mellitus harbor a glucokinase mutation, whereas at least one study found no glucokinase mutations in gestational diabetes mellitus patients. Pregnant women with MODY2 may require insulin therapy. Glucokinase is not believed to be a major genetic contributor to the development of type 2 diabetes.[55,162] Of interest, gain-of-function mutations in glucokinase can produce hyperinsulinemic neonatal hypoglycemia.[163,164]

MODY3: hepatocyte nuclear factor-1α

MODY3 (HNF-1α, chromosome 12q24.2) is the most common cause of MODY in the United Kingdom.[165] HNF-1α is expressed in liver and beta cells. HNF-4α regulates HNF-1α expression, providing a pathophysiologic link between MODY1 and MODY3.[166] HNF-4α regulates the expression of insulin (via HNF-1α), GLUT2 (glucose transporter-2), and other genes. Post-challenge elevations in plasma glucose levels are greater than elevations in fasting plasma glucose, which can even be found within the normal range in non-diabetic MODY3 carriers. Like MODY1, there is progressive insulinopenia with increasing age.[167] In the research studies, glucose priming increases insulin secretion.[168]

The clinical presentation of MODY3 is usually in adolescence or young adulthood. There is a favorable response to sulfonylurea therapy.[169] However approximately 1 in 3 MODY3 patients will eventually require insulin treatment. There can be a low renal threshold for glycosuria. Normal function of the HNF-1α gene is required *in utero*: infants born with an HNF-1α mutation are approx. 120 g lighter than their siblings. Complications in MODY3 patients can be observed (e.g., retinopathy). More than 65 HNF-1α mutations have been reported.[170] One estimate asserts that 1–2% of adult-onset cases of type 2 diabetes result from HNF-1α mutations.[150] Age at onset of disease and the family history appear to influence the frequency with which HNF-1α mutations are associated with type 2 diabetes.[60,61]

MODY4: insulin promoter factor-1

MODY4 was discovered in an infant with pancreatic agenesis who was small-for-gestational age, and displayed neonatal diabetes and exocrine pancreatic insufficiency.[171] The infant displayed homozygous insulin promoter factor-1 (IPF-1; chromosome 13q12.1) mutations. Upon study of the parents, both were shown to be carriers of the same mutation (e.g., heterozygotes). The father had type 2 diabetes and the mother had previously been diagnosed with gestational diabetes mellitus. Thorough review of the family histories revealed no evidence of consanguinity but a high frequency of diabetes on both sides of the family.

IPF-1 is also known as PDX-1 (pancreatic duodenal homeobox-1 protein), IDX-1 (islet duodenum homeobox-1), and STF-1 (Stefin A factor). IPF-1 regulates the expression of insulin, GLUT2, glucokinase, and other genes. Murine knockouts of IPF-1 and PTP-p48 produce pancreatic agenesis. The IPF-1 mutation that caused the initial report of MODY4 was a deletion of a cytosine (C) nucleotide at codon 63 that produced a subsequent frame shift mutation (Pro63fsdelC). A P33T mutation was later reported in Italian twins with early-onset type 2 diabetes.[172] Using a five-step hyperglycemic, clamp impaired insulin secretion and increased insulin sensitivity was identified in MODY4.[173]

Several studies have critically examined the possibility that MODY4 might be a significant cause of type 2 diabetes. In the United Kingdom, three IPF-1 mutations were found in MODY-X patients or patients with type 2 diabetes: C18R, D76N, and R197H.[172] Two of 12 MODY-X families (17%) had an IPF-1 mutation. Of 36 type 2 diabetes patients with disease onset before age 40, two had IPF-1 mutations (6%). Of 158 type 2 diabetes patients between the ages of 30 and 70 who had a diabetic sibling or parent, two had IPF-1 mutations (2.5%). In three of 192 French subjects with late-onset diabetes (6%), an InsCCG243 IPF-1 mutation was recognized.[174] Studies in Swedes with type 2 diabetes revealed three IPF-1 mutations: G212R, P239Q, and D76N. Of the early-onset Swedes, four of 115 (3.5%) had an IPF-1 mutation.[175] Of the late-onset Swedes, five of 183 (2.7%) had an IPF-1 mutation. However several other studies failed to detect IPF-1 mutations in the type 2 diabetes populations surveyed. No IPF-1 mutations were found in 40 Danes with MODY, 200 Danes with late-onset type 2 diabetes,[176] and only 1 IPF-1 mutation (C18R) was identified in 272 French subjects with late-onset type 2 diabetes (0.4%).[177]

MODY5: hepatocyte nuclear factor-1β

On screening Japanese MODY families lacking HNF-4α (MODY1), HNF-1α (MODY3), and IPF-1 (MODY4) mutations, researchers discovered MODY linkage to hepatocyte nuclear factor-1β (HNF-1β; chromosome 17).[178] Later, two European pedigrees were recognized with HNF-1β mutations.[179] Besides MODY, individuals with HNF-1β mutations can exhibit renal cysts, proteinuria, renal failure and, in females, vaginal aplasia, or rudimentary or bicornuate uterus.[180]

Presently, at least four HNF-1β mutations have been described: R177X, A263fsinsGG, P328L329fsdelCCTCT, and R137-K161del.[181] Acting as a transcription factor, HNF-1β can homodimerize or form heterodimers with HNF-1α. Because HNF-1β (MODY5) regulates HNF-4α (MODY1), there is an etiologic link between MODY5 and MODY1. MODY5 is a rare cause of MODY and none of 11 United Kingdom MODY-X families displayed HNF-1β mutations.[182] Rare HNF-1β mutations have been observed in type 2 diabetes subjects.[183]

MODY6: NeuroD1/Beta2

MODY6 was recently discovered in an Icelandic MODY family[184] when a missense E110K NeuroD1 mutation was found to be co-inherited with diabetes. An earlier report described one Europoid MODY family that exhibited a P206fsinsC NeuroD1 mutation.[185] However, NeuroD1 was not linked to diabetes in Japanese MODY pedigrees.[186] Another NeuroD1 mutation (R111L) was detected in one type 2 diabetes family characterized by obesity and hyperinsulinism.[74] Furthermore, NeuroD1 was not associated by linkage or mutational analysis with type 2 diabetes in France.[76]

NeuroD1, also known as Beta2, is a transcription factor that modulates insulin gene transcription.[187] NeuroD1 is detected in pancreatic endocrine cells, intestine, and brain. Secretin and cholecystokinin expression are dependent, in part, on NeuroD1. NeuroD1 can also induce neurons to differentiate. Concerning beta cells, the Beta2/NeuroD murine knockout reduces beta-cell number.[187]

MODY-X

'MODY-X' is a term applied to families that display clinical features of MODY but do not demonstrate a mutation in any of the genes so far recognized as causes of MODY. The key clinical feature in such families is autosomal dominant inheritance of youth-onset diabetes.[188] A 1999 paper from Doria *et al.*[189] reported 220 diabetic individuals from 29 families negative for MODY1 and MODY3 mutations. Surprisingly, there was evidence for insulin resistance in these pedigrees with insulin levels higher than in MODY3 subjects, therapeutic insulin doses higher than in MODY3, an approx. 50% prevalence of obesity, increased frequencies of elevated triglyceride and cholesterol levels, hypertension, and nephropathy. In contrast, four French MODY-X families[190] were not hyperinsulinemic. In Brazil, 58% of MODY pedigrees fall into the MODY-X category. The causes of ADM are largely unknown: Winter *et al.* reported a novel glucokinase mutation in one of 10 ADM families studied.[132] There is a growing list of transcription factors that have been examined that are not presently linked to MODY-X phenotypes (Table 11.6).[186,191–200]

Mitochondrial diabetes syndromes

Mitochondria are usually solely inherited from the mother.[201] Therefore, mitochondrial diseases are passed from affected mothers to their offspring.[202,203] The severity of the disorder depends upon the nature of the specific mitochondrial mutation, the proportion of mitochondria so

Table 11.6 Transcription factors not associated with MODY

Gene	Protein	Genomic location	MODY population studied
HNF3A	HNF-3α	14q12–q13	Japanese
HNF3B	HNF-3β	20p11	Japanese, French
HNF4G	HNF-4γ	8q	Japanese, US, and Canada
HNF6	HNF-6	15q21.1–q21.2	Japanese
NEUROD4	NeuroD4	12q13	Japanese
NEUROG3	Neurogenin 3	10q21.2–q21.3	Japanese, Danes
NKX2B	Nkx2.2	20p11	Japanese

affected (heteroplasmy), and the distribution of the abnormal mitochondria among tissues. Normally there are 6–10 copies of the 16,569 base pair mitochondrial genome per mitochondrion and cells can have 100s to 1000s of mitochondria.[204]

Mutations in the mitochondrial genome can interfere with cellular energy generation.[205] This is consistent with the role of the mitochondrion as the 'powerhouse' of the cell where beta oxidation of fatty acids, the Krebs cycle, and oxidative phosphorylation take place.[206] The organs most susceptible to dysfunction when energy production is deficient are organs that exhibit high metabolic rates: the nervous system, the heart, and skeletal muscle.[207] In addition, mitochondrial diseases can affect the beta cell, causing insulinopenia. Most cases of 'mitochondrial' diabetes present clinically as non-insulin dependent diabetes[208] but rare patients with mitochondrial mutations have had a type-1-diabetes-like phenotype[209] with islet autoantibodies.[210] Mitochondrial diabetes has been reported in children as young as age 10.[211] Mitochondrial diabetes may cause 1–3% of cases of phenotypic type 2 diabetes in Japanese adults. Like MODY, mitochondrial diabetes is classified as a genetic defect of the beta-cell function under the heading of 'other specific types of diabetes' because of insulinopenia.[212]

Mitochondrial diabetes may appear as the only manifestation of a mitochondrial mutation or may exist as part of a multisystem disease complex associated with deafness, hypertrophic cardiomyopathy, Leber's hereditary optic neuropathy (LHON), MERRF (mitochondrial encephalo-myopathy, myoclonus epilepsy, ragged-red fibers, and sensorineural hearing loss), or MELAS (myopathy, encephalopathy, lactic acidosis, and stroke-like syndrome).[213] The most common mitochondrial mutation associated with diabetes is A3243G affecting tRNA$^{Leu(UUR)}$. The A3243G mutation can occur in isolation or associated with other mitochondrial mutations.

The A3243G mutation can cause diabetes alone or diabetes plus deafness or diabetes as part of MELAS. Hypertrophic cardiomyopathy and diabetes in association with the A3243G mutation occur with the following coincident mutations: C946A in 12SrRNA, A1041G in 12SrRNA, T3394C in NADH dehydrogenase subunit 1 (ND1), G4491A in NADH dehydrogenase subunit 2 (ND2), and G11963A in NADH dehydrogenase subunit 4 (ND4). The following mutations can produce mitochondrial diabetes and are not associated with a coexistent A3243G mutation: A3252G (tRNA$^{Leu(UUR)}$), C3256T (tRNA$^{Leu(UUR)}$), A3260G (tRNA$^{Leu(UUR)}$), T3271C (tRNA$^{Leu(UUR)}$), G3316A (ND1), A8344G (tRNA^{Lys}), and T14709C (tRNA^{Glu}). These later mutations are usually associated with skeletal myopathy and, less commonly, cardiomyopathy, LHON, or MERRF.

Other specific types of diabetes

Except for the lipodystrophies, these 'other specific types of diabetes' will be classified and discussed according to their mode of inheritance. Some genetic causes of diabetes occur sporadically such as McCune–Albright syndrome (G protein mutations) or Sotos's syndrome (NSD1 mutations). There are many, many forms of diabetes previously referred to as 'secondary' diabetes.

Autosomal dominant disorders associated with non-MODY diabetes

Diabetes can occur secondary to pheochromocytoma that is part of *multiple endocrine neoplasia type 2* (MEN2). MEN2 is inherited as an autosomal dominant. Mutations in the RET proto-oncogene (chromosome 10q11.2) produce MEN2.[214] *MEN1* can produce diabetes via the development of Cushing disease, acromegaly, glucagonoma, or somatostatinoma.[215] MEN1 results from loss-of-heterozygosity for a tumor suppressor gene (MEN1) on chromosome 11q13. Rarely, pheochromocytoma can be inherited as an autosomal dominant independent of MEN2.[216]

Other autosomal dominant disorders where diabetes or abnormal glucose tolerance has been described include achondroplasia, Bannayan–Riley–Ruvalcaba syndrome (*PTEN* gene, chromosome 10q23), Steinert myotonic dystrophy syndrome (a triple-repeat expansion disease, chromosome 19q13.3), acute intermittent porphyria (chromosome 11q23.3), and insulinopathies and hyperproinsulinemias (insulin gene, chromosome 11p15.5). Although a genetic disease, Huntington's disease (chromosome 4p16.3) does not manifest until adulthood.

Codominant or recessive forms of diabetes

Deletions or loss-of-function genetic defects in the *insulin receptor* can cause severe insulin-resistant diabetes.[217] Acanthosis nigricans and hyperandrogenism (in females) are usually observed in individuals who suffer from insulin receptor mutations. When these features and insulin-resistant diabetes are the expression of the insulin receptor mutation, the patient is diagnosed with 'type A insulin resistance.' In contrast, antagonistic insulin receptor autoantibodies produce 'type B insulin resistance.'

Generally, subjects bearing two mutant insulin receptor gene alleles are more insulin-resistant than subjects with a single mutant allele. For example, heterozygosity for an insulin receptor mutation can present clinically as type 2 diabetes, whereas homozygosity or compound heterozygosity can produce a very severe phenotype such as leprechaunism (Donohue syndrome) or Rabson–Mendenhall syndrome where the metabolic derangement is of intermediate severity.[218,219] Infants with leprechaunism exhibit severe growth failure of prenatal onset, prenatal adipose tissue deficiency, full lips, islet cell hyperplasia (in response to severe insulin resistance), hirsutism, enlargement of the breasts and labia, and usually die within the first year of life. Children with Rabson–Mendenhall syndrome display short stature, abnormal teeth and nails, and hyperplasia of the pineal gland.

Autosomal recessive forms of diabetes

Cystic fibrosis

Diabetes is a component of many inherited conditions. For example, with increasing duration of disease, an insulinopenic form of diabetes becomes more prevalent in individuals with cystic fibrosis.[220] Located on chromosome 7q31.2, mutations in the cystic fibrosis transmembrane conductance regulator (CFTR) gene cause cystic fibrosis. Approximately 70% of CFTR allele mutations involve a deletion of the phenylalanine codon at residue 508.

Wolfram syndrome

Wolfram syndrome is a rare autosomal recessive disorder that is characterized by diabetes insipidus, diabetes mellitus, optic atrophy, and deafness ('DIDMOAD' syndrome). Other neurologic symptoms include ataxia, myoclonus, peripheral neuropathy, and psychiatric illness.[221] Wolfram syndrome is caused by mutations in the WFS1 gene located on chromosome 4p16.[222] The WFS1 gene is 33.4 kilobases in length, has 8 exons, and predicts a transmembrane protein of 890 amino acids with an apparent molecular mass of 100 kDa. Hydrophilic amino and carboxy termini are separated by a hydrophobic region comprising nine predicted transmembrane segments. Biochemical analysis demonstrated that the WFS1 protein is an integral, endoglycosidase H-sensitive membrane glycoprotein with expression primarily in the endoplasmic reticulum.[223] Of interest, non-inactivating mutations in WFS1 are responsible for autosomal-dominant inherited, non-syndromic low-frequency hearing impairment.[224] There is preliminary evidence that WFS1 may serve as a type 2 diabetes susceptibility gene in the general population.[225]

Werner syndrome

Werner syndrome is characterized by a premature-aging-like phenotype of cataracts, thin skin with thick fibrous subcutaneous tissue, and gray sparse hair. Inherited as an autosomal recessive, the Werner syndrome gene (WRN) has been mapped to chromosome 8p12 and encodes a DNA helicase. One report describes insulin resistance in subjects with Werner syndrome.[226] Non-insulin dependent diabetes can also occur in *Bloom syndrome* (short stature, malar hypoplasia, telangiectasia, and facial erythema). Bloom syndrome results from a mutation in the BLM gene (chromosome 15q26.1) that also acts as a helicase. There is an increased risk for cancer in both Werner's syndrome and Bloom syndrome.[227]

Bardet–Biedl syndrome

Bardet–Biedl syndrome is inherited as an autosomal recessive and is characterized by retinitis pigmentosa, polydactyly, obesity, hypogonadism, mental deficiency, and renal impairment.[228] Bardet–Biedl syndrome (also known as Lawrence–Moon–Biedl syndrome) is genetically heterogeneous, involving at least six loci.[229]

Autoimmune polyglandular syndrome I (APS I)

APS I is an autosomal recessive disorder mapped to the AIRE (autoimmune regulator) gene on chromosome 21q22.3.[230] Approximately 10% of patients with APS I will develop type 1 diabetes. Although autoimmune in etiology, APS I is mentioned because this disorder has a clear Mendelian mode of inheritance.

Hereditary hemochromatosis

Hereditary hemochromatosis results from mutations in the *HFE* gene located within the human leukocyte antigen complex (HLA) on the short arm of chromosome 6 at 6p21.3.[231] Whereas children may display cardiomyopathy and gonadal insufficiency, adults are more likely to develop liver disease and diabetes mellitus (e.g., bronze diabetes).[232] Diabetes in this autosomal recessive condition results from iron-induced beta-cell dysfunction, producing reduced insulin secretion as well as insulin resistance from hepatic disease. Some patients may show elevated insulin levels secondary to depressed hepatic clearance of insulin. In contrast to type 1 diabetes where the islets are depleted of beta cells and type 2 diabetes where 50% of autopsy cases display amyloid deposition, in hemochromatosis the islets are of normal shape and size. Because *thalassemia* can also cause iron overload and beta-cell damage, thalassemia major is another potential cause of autosomal recessive diabetes.

Other autosomal recessive disorders

Other autosomal recessive disorders where diabetes or abnormal glucose tolerance has been described include ataxia telangectasia syndrome (Louis–Bar syndrome, gene: ATM serine–threonine kinase, chromosome 11q22.3), Johanson–Blizzard syndrome (unmapped at present), alpha-1-antitrypsin deficiency (chromosome 14q32.1), glycogen storage disease type I (chromosome 17q21), Friedreich ataxia (chromosome 9q13-q21.1), and Cockayne syndrome (chromosome 5). Diabetes does not necessarily appear in childhood in these conditions.

Gene imprinting defects associated with diabetes

Diabetes can be observed in children affected with *Prader–Willi syndrome*. Surprisingly, despite their extreme morbid obesity, most Prader–Willi children do not demonstrate insulin resistance and their diabetes is insulinopenic in nature.[233,234] Prader–Willi syndrome results from defective imprinting of paternal genes located on chromosome 15q11–13. Some cases of Prader–Willi syndrome alternatively result from uniparental maternal disomy.

Chromosomal disorders associated with diabetes

Diabetes is increased in frequency in individuals with Down syndrome, Klinefelter syndrome, or Turner syndrome. Usually the diabetes is autoimmune in etiology (type 1a diabetes). Although such cases do not fall into the category of non-autoimmune childhood diabetes, these associations are mentioned because the individuals are affected with an underlying genetic (chromosomal) disorder. Partial or complete uniparental disomy of chromosome 6 can cause neonatal diabetes.[235]

Lipodystrophies

Because of their shared phenotype of generalized or localized absence or loss of adipose tissue, severe insulin resistance, and type 2 diabetes, the lipodystrophies will be reviewed as a group as opposed to classification by their mode of inheritance. Whereas lipodystrophy can be acquired (e.g., generalized, partial, localized, or secondary to protease inhibitors used in the treatment of human immunodeficiency virus infection), there are several forms of inherited lipodystrophy: congenital generalized, familial partial-Dunnigan type, familial partial-mandibuloacral dysplasia type, and familial partial-Kobberling type.[236] Congenital generalized lipodystrophy (CGL; Berardinelli–Seip syndrome) is inherited as an autosomal recessive trait that can be caused by defects in two different genes. Mutations in the *AGPAT2* gene on chromosome 9q34 encoding 1-acylglycerol-3-phosphate O-acyltransferase can cause CGL.[237] Alternatively, mutations in the *BSCL2* gene (Berardinelli–Seip congenital lipodystrophy 2) can also cause CGL.[238]

Familial partial lipodystrophy – Dunnigan variety (FPLD) is inherited as an autosomal dominant. Mutations in the *lamin A/C* (LMNA) gene on the chromosome 1q21–22 cause FPLD.[239] In FPLD, fat may be absent from some subcutaneous areas only to be increased in other areas. Autosomal recessive familial partial lipodystrophy – mandibuloacral dysplasia (FPL–MAD) involves a maldeveloped jaw, producing dental crowding, underdeveloped clavicles, and resorption of terminal phalanges in association with short stature. The molecular defect is unknown at present. The mode of transmission of familial partial lipodystrophy – Kobberling variety – is unclear. In this condition there is loss of fat in the extremities. The *peroxisome proliferator-activated receptor gamma* (PPARG) gene on chromosome 3p25 is a candidate gene in this disorder.[240]

Clinical application of genetics in the practice of pediatric diabetology

Understanding the genetic basis of a disease can foster the development of novel and more effective therapies. When a disorder is inherited, family members can be screened metabolically or even genetically for the presence of diabetes or predilection to diabetes. This affords an opportunity for prevention. The daily management of diabetes is also greatly influenced by the type of diabetes affecting an individual. To this end, by taking a thorough family history and appreciating the clinical characteristics of the diabetic state affecting the proband, assessment of the mode of inheritance of diabetes can greatly assist in the classification of the patient's disease. With special reference to the genetics of non-autoimmune diabetes, the following clinical approach is suggested. Other authors have provided similar approaches.[241]

Diagnosis of diabetes

Nonketotic obese diabetic children with a family history of maternally transmitted diabetes are identified as having mitochondrial diabetes. Further supportive evidence of mitochondrial diabetes includes the coexistence of deafness or impaired hearing, skeletal muscle myopathy, and cardiomyopathy or neurologic disorders (e.g., seizures, encephalopathy). If the nonketotic obese child has a parent with non-insulin-dependent diabetes onset before age 25, MODY is likely.[242] In the case of African-American children with suspected ADM, the age of onset of diabetes in the parents can be extended up to 40 years old. The nonketotic lean child with a history of maternally inherited diabetes is affected with mitochondrial diabetes. Finally, nonketotic lean diabetic children with a parent with non-insulin-dependent diabetes onset before age 25 are diagnosed with MODY.

Routine laboratory testing for mitochondrial mutations and MODY mutations is not readily available. There are specialty laboratories in the United States that focus on mitochondrial diagnosis. In addition, at least one laboratory in the United Kingdom (Molecular Genetics Laboratory at the Royal Devon & Exeter NHS Healthcare Trust; http://www.ex.ac.uk/diabetesgenes/mody/diagnostic/) offers testing for glucokinase, HNF-1α, and HNF-4α mutations. Various research laboratories have invested heavily in the study of MODY or mitochondrial diabetes syndromes: however, the clinician generally remains dependent on history taking and investigative skills to solve diagnostic dilemmas. In summary, the basic and essential process of taking a thorough family history can provide substantial diagnostic information when the etiology of diabetes in a child or adolescent is not straightforward. Understanding the genetics of non-autoimmune diabetes will certainly influence the future care of children and the prediction of disease.

References

1. Froguel P, Velho G. Genetic determinants of type 2 diabetes. *Recent Prog Horm Res* 2001; **56**:91–105.
2. Rotter JI, Vadheim CM, Rimoin DL. Diabetes mellitus. In: King RA, Rotter JI, Motulsky AG, eds. *The Genetic Basis of Common Diseases.* New York: Oxford University Press, 1992: 413–18.
3. Kyvik KO, Green A, Beck-Nielsen H. Concordance rates of insulin dependent diabetes mellitus: a population based study of young Danish twins. *BMJ* 1995; **311**(7010):913–17.
4. Pani MA, Badenhoop K. Digging the genome for diabetes mellitus: the 2nd ADA Research Symposium on the Genetics of Diabetes, San Jose, CA, USA, 17–19 October 1999. *Trends Endocrinol Metab* 2000; **11**(4):148–50.
5. Glaser N, Jones KL. Non-insulin dependent diabetes mellitus in children and adolescents. *Adv Pediatr* 1996; **43**:359–96.
6. Pinhas-Hamiel O, Dolan LM, Daniels SR. Increased incidence of non-insulin dependent diabetes mellitus among adolescents. *J Pediatr* 1996; **128**:608–15.
7. Glaser NS. Non-insulin dependent diabetes mellitus in childhood and adolescence. *Pediatr Clin N Am* 1997; **44**(2):307–37.
8. Jones KL. Non-insulin dependent diabetes in children and adolescents: the therapeutic challenge. *Clin Pediatr* 1998; **2**:103–10.
9. Hanson RL, Pettitt DJ, Bennett PH *et al*. Familial relationships between obesity and NIDDM. *Diabetes* 1995; **44**(4):418–22.
10. Kuczmarski RJ, Flegal KM, Campbell SM, Johnson CL. Increasing prevalence of overweight among US adults. The National Health and Nutrition Examination Surveys, 1960 to 1991. *JAMA* 1994; **272**(3):205–11.
11. Ford ES, Giles WH, Dietz WH. Prevalence of the metabolic syndrome among US adults: findings from the Third National Health and Nutrition Examination Survey. *JAMA* 2002; **287**(3):356–9.
12. Moller DE, Bjorbaek C, Vidal-Puig A. Candidate genes for insulin resistance. *Diabetes Care* 1996; **19**(4):396–400.
13. Stern MP, Mitchell BD. Genetics of insulin resistance. In: Reaven GM, Laws A, eds. *Insulin Resistance: The Metabolic Syndrome.* Totowa, NJ, Humana Press, 1999:3–18.
14. Norman RA, Thompson DB, Foroud T *et al*. Genomewide search for genes influencing percent body fat in Pima Indians: suggestive linkage at chromosome 11q21–q22. Pima Diabetes Gene Group. *Am J Hum Genet* 1997; **60**(1):166–73.
15. Hager J, Dina C, Francke S *et al*. A genome-wide scan for human obesity genes reveals a major susceptibility locus on chromosome 10. *Nat Genet* 1998; **20**(3):304–8.
16. Mitchell BD, Cole SA, Comuzzie AG *et al*. A quantitative trait locus influencing BMI maps to the region of the beta-3 adrenergic receptor. *Diabetes* 1999; **48**(9):1863–7.
17. Lee JH, Reed DR, Li WD *et al*. Genome scan for human obesity and linkage to markers in 20q13. *Am J Hum Genet* 1999; **64**(1):196–209.
18. van der Kallen CJ, Cantor RM, van Greevenbroek MM *et al*. Genome scan for adiposity in Dutch dyslipidemic families reveals novel quantitative trait

loci for leptin, body mass index and soluble tumor necrosis factor receptor superfamily 1A. *Int J Obes Relat Metab Disord* 2000; **24**(11):1381–91.

19. Hinney A, Ziegler A, Oeffner F *et al.* Independent confirmation of a major locus for obesity on chromosome 10. *J Clin Endocrinol Metab* 2000; **85**(8):2962–5.

20. Ohman M, Oksanen L, Kaprio J *et al.* Genome-wide scan of obesity in Finnish sibpairs reveals linkage to chromosome Xq24. *J Clin Endocrinol Metab* 2000; **85**(9):3183–90.

21. Perola M, Ohman M, Hiekkalinna T *et al.* Quantitative-trait-locus analysis of body-mass index and of stature, by combined analysis of genome scans of five Finnish study groups. *Am J Hum Genet* 2001; **69**(1):117–23.

22. Feitosa MF, Borecki IB, Rich SS *et al.* Quantitative-trait loci influencing body-mass index reside on chromosomes 7 and 13: the National Heart, Lung, and Blood Institute Family Heart Study. *Am J Hum Genet* 2002; **70**(1):72–82.

23. Arner P. Obesity – a genetic disease of adipose tissue? *Br J Nutr* 2000; **83**(suppl 1):S9–16.

24. Engert JC, Vohl MC, Williams SM *et al.* 5′ flanking variants of resistin are associated with obesity. *Diabetes* 2002; **51**(5):1629–34.

25. Valve R, Sivenius K, Miettinen R *et al.* Two polymorphisms in the peroxi-some proliferator-activated receptor-gamma gene are associated with severe overweight among obese women. *J Clin Endocrinol Metab* 1999; **84**(10):3708–12.

26. del Giudice EM, Santoro N, Cirillo G *et al.* Mutational screening of the CART gene in obese children: identifying a mutation (Leu34Phe) associated with reduced resting energy expenditure and cosegregating with obesity phenotype in a large family. *Diabetes* 2001; **50**(9):2157–60.

27. Oizumi T, Daimon M, Saitoh T *et al.* Genotype Arg/Arg, but not Trp/Arg, of the Trp64Arg polymorphism of the beta(3)-adrenergic receptor is associated with type 2 diabetes and obesity in a large Japanese sample. *Diabetes Care* 2001; **24**(9):1579–83.

28. Menzaghi C, Ercolino T, Di Paola R *et al.* A haplotype at the adiponectin locus is associated with obesity and other features of the insulin resistance syndrome. *Diabetes* 2002; **51**(7):2306–12.

29. Chouchane L, Danguir J, Beji C *et al.* Genetic variation in the stress protein hsp70–2 gene is highly associated with obesity. *Int J Obes Relat Metab Disord* 2001; **25**(4):462–6.

30. Halsall DJ, Luan J, Saker P *et al.* Uncoupling protein 3 genetic variants in human obesity: the c-55t promoter polymorphism is negatively correlated with body mass index in a UK Caucasian population. *Int J Obes Relat Metab Disord* 2001; **25**(4):472–7.

31. Clement K, Dina C, Basdevant A *et al.* A sib-pair analysis study of 15 candi-date genes in French families with morbid obesity: indication for linkage with islet 1 locus on chromosome 5q. *Diabetes* 1999; **48**(2):398–402.

32. Abney M, Ober C, McPeek MS. Quantitative-trait homozygosity and associa-tion mapping and empirical genomewide significance in large, complex pedigrees: fasting serum-insulin level in the Hutterites. *Am J Hum Genet* 2002; **70**(4):920–34.

33. Xiang KS, Cox NJ, Sanz N *et al.* Insulin-receptor and apolipoprotein genes contribute to development of NIDDM in Chinese Americans. *Diabetes* 1989; **38**(1):17–23.

34. Houlston RS, Snowden C, Laker MF *et al.* Variation in the apolipoprotein B gene and development of type 2 diabetes mellitus. *Dis Markers* 1991; **9**(2):87–96.

35. Yamada K, Ishiyama-Shigemoto S, Ichikawa F *et al.* Polymorphism in the 5'-leader cistron of the beta2-adrenergic receptor gene associated with obesity and type 2 diabetes. *J Clin Endocrinol Metab* 1999; **84**(5):1754–7.

36. Kondo H, Shimomura I, Matsukawa Y *et al.* Association of adiponectin mutation with type 2 diabetes: a candidate gene for the insulin resistance syndrome. *Diabetes* 2002; **51**(7):2325–8.

37. Du W, Sun H, Wang H *et al.* Confirmation of susceptibility gene loci on chromosome 1 in northern China Han families with type 2 diabetes. *Chin Med J (Engl)* 2001; **114**(8):876–8.

38. Elbein SC, Bragg KL, Hoffman MD *et al.* Linkage studies of NIDDM with 23 chromosome 11 markers in a sample of whites of northern European descent. *Diabetes* 1996; **45**(3):370–5.

39. Klannemark M, Orho M, Langin D *et al.* The putative role of the hormone-sensitive lipase gene in the pathogenesis of type II diabetes mellitus and abdominal obesity. *Diabetologia* 1998; **41**(12):1516–22.

40. Schwanstecher C, Meyer U, Schwanstecher M. K(IR)6.2 polymorphism predisposes to type 2 diabetes by inducing overactivity of pancreatic beta-cell ATP-sensitive K(+) channels. *Diabetes* 2002; **51**(3):875–9.

41. Marion E, Kaisaki PJ, Pouillon V *et al.* The gene INPPL1, encoding the lipid phosphatase SHIP2, is a candidate for type 2 diabetes in rat and man. *Diabetes* 2002; **51**(7):2012–17.

42. Hani el-H, Zouali H, Philippi A *et al.* Indication for genetic linkage of the phosphoenolpyruvate carboxykinase (PCK1) gene region on chromosome 20q to non-insulin-dependent diabetes mellitus. *Diabetes Metab* 1996; **22**(6):451–4.

43. Zouali H, Hani EH, Philippi A *et al.* A susceptibility locus for early-onset non-insulin dependent (type 2) diabetes mellitus maps to chromosome 20q, proximal to the phosphoenolpyruvate carboxykinase gene. *Hum Mol Genet* 1997; **6**(9):1401–8.

44. Lindgren CM, Hirshhorn JN. The genetics of type 2 diabetes. *The Endocrinologist* 2001; **11**:178–87.

45. Yoshida H, Ohagi S, Sanke T *et al.* Association of the prohormone convertase 2 gene (PCSK2) on chromosome 20 with NIDDM in Japanese subjects. *Diabetes* 1995; **44**(4):389–93.

46. Mitchell BD, Cole SA, Comuzzie AG *et al.* A quantitative trait locus influencing BMI maps to the region of the beta-3 adrenergic receptor. *Diabetes* 1999; **48**(9):1863–7.

47. Buettner R, Schaffler A, Arndt H *et al.* The Trp64Arg polymorphism of the beta 3-adrenergic receptor gene is not associated with obesity or type 2 diabetes mellitus in a large population-based Caucasian cohort. *J Clin Endocrinol Metab* 1998; **83**(8):2892–7.

48. Vionnet N, Hani EH, Lesage S *et al.* Genetics of NIDDM in France: studies with 19 candidate genes in affected sib pairs. *Diabetes* 1997; **46**(6):1062–8.

49. Elbein SC, Hoffman MD, Mayorga RA *et al*. Do non-insulin-dependent diabetes mellitus (NIDDM) and insulin-dependent diabetes mellitus (IDDM) share genetic susceptibility loci? An analysis of putative IDDM susceptibility regions in familial NIDDM. *Metabolism* 1997; **46**(1):48–52.

50. Frayling TM, McCarthy MI, Walker M *et al*. No evidence for linkage at candidate type 2 diabetes susceptibility loci on chromosomes 12 and 20 in United Kingdom Caucasians. *J Clin Endocrinol Metab* 2000; **85**(2):853–7.

51. Hager J, Hansen L, Vaisse C *et al*. A missense mutation in the glucagon receptor gene is associated with non-insulin-dependent diabetes mellitus. *Nat Genet* 1995; **9**(3):299–304.

52. Odawara M, Tachi Y, Yamashita K. Absence of association between the Gly40→Ser mutation in the human glucagon receptor and Japanese patients with non-insulin-dependent diabetes mellitus or impaired glucose tolerance. *Hum Genet* 1996; **98**(6):636–9.

53. Chiu KC, Province MA, Dowse GK *et al*. A genetic marker at the glucokinase gene locus for type 2 (non-insulin-dependent) diabetes mellitus in Mauritian Creoles. *Diabetologia* 1992; **35**(7):632–8.

54. Noda K, Matsutani A, Tanizawa Y *et al*. Polymorphic microsatellite repeat markers at the glucokinase gene locus are positively associated with NIDDM in Japanese. *Diabetes* 1993; **42**(8):1147–52.

55. Chiu KC, Tanizawa Y, Permutt MA. Glucokinase gene variants in the common form of NIDDM. *Diabetes* 1993; **42**(4):579–82.

56. Alcolado JC, Baroni MG, Li SR. Association between a restriction fragment length polymorphism at the liver/islet cell (GluT 2) glucose transporter and familial type 2 (non-insulin-dependent) diabetes mellitus. *Diabetologia* 1991; **34**(10):734–6.

57. Oelbaum RS. Analysis of three glucose transporter genes in a Caucasian population: no associations with non-insulin-dependent diabetes and obesity. *Clin Genet* 1992; **42**(5):260–6.

58. Groop LC, Kankuri M, Schalin-Jantti C *et al*. Association between polymorphism of the glycogen synthase gene and non-insulin-dependent diabetes mellitus. *N Engl J Med* 1993; **328**(1):10–14.

59. Bjorbaek C, Echwald SM, Hubricht P *et al*. Genetic variants in promoters and coding regions of the muscle glycogen synthase and the insulin-responsive GLUT4 genes in NIDDM. *Diabetes* 1994; **43**(8):976–83.

60. Elbein SC, Teng K, Yount P, Scroggin E. Linkage and molecular scanning analyses of MODY3/hepatocyte nuclear factor-1 alpha gene in typical familial type 2 diabetes: evidence for novel mutations in exons 8 and 10. *J Clin Endocrinol Metab* 1998; **83**(6):2059–65.

61. Lesage S, Hani EH, Philippi A *et al*. Linkage analyses of the MODY3 locus on chromosome 12q with late-onset NIDDM. *Diabetes* 1995; **44**(10):1243–7.

62. Zhu Q, Yamagata K, Yu L *et al*. Identification of missense mutations in the hepatocyte nuclear factor-3beta gene in Japanese subjects with late-onset type II diabetes mellitus. *Diabetologia* 2000; **43**(9):1197–200.

63. Bowden DW, Sale M, Howard TD *et al*. Linkage of genetic markers on human chromosomes 20 and 12 to NIDDM in Caucasian sib pairs with a history of diabetic nephropathy. *Diabetes* 1997; **46**(5):882–6.

64. Malecki MT, Antonellis A, Casey P *et al*. Exclusion of the hepatocyte nuclear factor 4alpha as a candidate gene for late-onset NIDDM linked with chromosome 20q. *Diabetes* 1998; **47**(6):970–2.

65. Rotwein P, Chyn R, Chirgwin J *et al*. Polymorphism in the 5′-flanking region of the human insulin gene and its possible relation to type 2 diabetes. *Science* 1981; **213**(4512):1117–20.

66. Elbein SC, Corsetti L, Goldgar D *et al*. Insulin gene in familial NIDDM. Lack of linkage in Utah Mormon pedigrees. *Diabetes* 1988; **37**(5):569–76.

67. Raboudi SH, Mitchell BD, Stern MP *et al*. Type II diabetes mellitus and polymorphism of insulin-receptor gene in Mexican Americans. *Diabetes* 1989; **38**(8):975–80.

68. Cox NJ, Epstein PA, Spielman RS. Linkage studies on NIDDM and the insulin and insulin-receptor genes. *Diabetes* 1989; **38**(5):653–8.

69. Stern MP, Mitchell BD, Blangero J *et al*. Evidence for a major gene for type II diabetes and linkage analyses with selected candidate genes in Mexican-Americans. *Diabetes* 1996; **45**(5):563–8.

70. Sigal RJ, Doria A, Warram JH, Krolewski AS. Codon 972 polymorphism in the insulin receptor substrate-1 gene, obesity, and risk of noninsulin-dependent diabetes mellitus. *J Clin Endocrinol Metab* 1996; **81**(4):1657–9.

71. Sakagashira S, Sanke T, Hanabusa T *et al*. Missense mutation of amylin gene (S20G) in Japanese NIDDM patients. *Diabetes* 1996; **45**(9):1279–81.

72. Gambino V, Menzel S, Trabb JB *et al*. An approach for identifying simple sequence repeat DNA polymorphisms near cloned cDNAs and genes. Linkage studies of the islet amyloid polypeptide/amylin and liver glycogen synthase genes and NIDDM. *Diabetes* 1996; **45**(3):291–4.

73. Shimomura H, Sanke T, Hanabusa T *et al*. Nonsense mutation of islet-1 gene (Q310X) found in a type 2 diabetic patient with a strong family history. *Diabetes* 2000; **49**(9):1597–600.

74. Malecki MT, Jhala US, Antonellis A *et al*. Mutations in NEUROD1 are associated with the development of type 2 diabetes mellitus. *Nat Genet* 1999; **23**(3):323–8.

75. Shimajiri Y, Sanke T, Furuta H *et al*. A missense mutation of Pax4 gene (R121W) is associated with type 2 diabetes in Japanese. *Diabetes* 2001; **50**(12):2864–9.

76. Dupont S, Vionnet N, Chevre JC *et al*. No evidence of linkage or diabetes-associated mutations in the transcription factors BETA2/NEUROD1 and PAX4 in Type II diabetes in France. *Diabetologia* 1999; **42**(4):480–4.

77. Reynet C, Kahn CR. Rad: a member of the Ras family overexpressed in muscle of type II diabetic humans. *Science* 1993; **262**(5138):1441–4.

78. Orho M, Carlsson M, Kanninen T, Groop LC. Polymorphism at the rad gene is not associated with NIDDM in Finns. *Diabetes* 1996; **45**(4):429–33.

79. Chen YH, Hansen L, Chen MX *et al*. Sequence of the human glycogen-associated regulatory subunit of type 1 protein phosphatase and analysis of its coding region and mRNA level in muscle from patients with NIDDM. *Diabetes* 1994; **43**(10):1234–41.

80. Inoue H, Ferrer J, Welling CM *et al*. Sequence variants in the sulfonylurea receptor (SUR) gene are associated with NIDDM in Caucasians. *Diabetes* 1996; **45**(6):825–31.

81. Inoue H, Ferrer J, Warren-Perry M *et al*. Sequence variants in the pancreatic islet beta-cell inwardly rectifying K+ channel Kir6.2 (Bir) gene: identification and lack of role in Caucasian patients with NIDDM. *Diabetes* 1997; **46**(3):502–7.

82. Hanis CL, Boerwinkle E, Chakraborty R *et al*. A genome-wide search for human non-insulin-dependent (type 2) diabetes genes reveals a major susceptibility locus on chromosome 2. *Nat Genet* 1996; **13**(2):161–6.

83. Hani EH, Hager J, Philippi A *et al*. Mapping NIDDM susceptibility loci in French families: studies with markers in the region of NIDDM1 on chromosome 2q. *Diabetes* 1997; **46**(7):1225–6.

84. Ciccarese M, Tonolo G, Delin I *et al*. Preliminary data on a genome search in NIDDM siblings: the NIDDM1 locus on chromosome 2 is not linked to NIDDM in the Sardinian population. Study Group for the Genetics of Diabetes in Sardinia. *Diabetologia* 1997; **40**(11):1366–7.

85. Ghosh S, Hauser ER, Magnuson VL *et al*. A large sample of Finnish diabetic sib-pairs reveals no evidence for a non-insulin-dependent diabetes mellitus susceptibility locus at 2qter. *J Clin Invest* 1998; **102**(4):704–9.

86. Cox NJ, Frigge M, Nicolae DL *et al*. Loci on chromosomes 2 (NIDDM1) and 15 interact to increase susceptibility to diabetes in Mexican Americans. *Nat Genet* 1999; **21**(2):213–15.

87. Horikawa Y, Oda N, Cox NJ *et al*. Genetic variation in the gene encoding calpain-10 is associated with type 2 diabetes mellitus. *Nat Genet* 2000; **26**(2):163–75.

88. Altshuler D, Daly M, Kruglyak L. Guilt by association. *Nat Genet* 2000; **26**(2):135–7.

89. Permutt MA, Bernal-Mizrachi E, Inoue H. Calpain 10: the first positional cloning of a gene for type 2 diabetes? *J Clin Invest* 2000; **106**(7):819–21.

90. Fingerlin TE, Erdos MR, Watanabe RM *et al*. Variation in three single nucleotide polymorphisms in the calpain-10 gene not associated with type 2 diabetes in a large Finnish cohort. *Diabetes* 2002; **51**(5):1644–8.

91. Evans JC, Frayling TM, Cassell PG *et al*. Studies of association between the gene for calpain-10 and type 2 diabetes mellitus in the United Kingdom. *Am J Hum Genet* 2001; **69**(3):544–52.

92. Tsai HJ, Sun G, Weeks DE *et al*. Type 2 diabetes and three calpain-10 gene polymorphisms in Samoans: no evidence of association. *Am J Hum Genet* 2001; **69**(6):1236–44.

93. Hegele RA, Harris SB, Zinman B *et al*. Absence of association of type 2 diabetes with CAPN10 and PC-1 polymorphisms in Oji-Cree. *Diabetes Care* 2001; **24**(8):1498–9.

94. Elbein SC, Chu W, Ren Q *et al*. Role of calpain-10 gene variants in familial type 2 diabetes in Caucasians. *J Clin Endocrinol Metab* 2002; **87**(2):650–4.

95. Cassell PG, Jackson AE, North BV *et al*. Haplotype combinations of calpain 10 gene polymorphisms associate with increased risk of impaired glucose tolerance and type 2 diabetes in South Indians. *Diabetes* 2002; **51**(5): 1622–8.

96. Garant MJ, Kao WH, Brancati F *et al*. SNP43 of CAPN10 and the risk of type 2 diabetes in African-Americans: the Atherosclerosis Risk in Communities Study. *Diabetes* 2002; **51**(1):231–7.

97. Malecki MT, Moczulski DK, Klupa T *et al*. Homozygous combination of calpain 10 gene haplotypes is associated with type 2 diabetes mellitus in a Polish population. *Eur J Endocrinol* 2002; **146**(5):695–9.
98. Hinney A, Antwerpen B, Geller F *et al*. No evidence for involvement of the calpain-10 gene 'high-risk' haplotype combination for non-insulin-dependent diabetes mellitus in early onset obesity. *Mol Genet Metab* 2002; **76**(2):152–6.
99. Fullerton SM, Bartoszewicz A, Ybazeta G *et al*. Geographic and haplotype structure of candidate type 2 diabetes susceptibility variants at the calpain-10 locus. *Am J Hum Genet* 2002; **70**(5):1096–106.
100. Cox NJ. Challenges in identifying genetic variation affecting susceptibility to type 2 diabetes: examples from studies of the calpain-10 gene. *Hum Mol Genet* 2001; **10**(20):2301–5.
101. Baier LJ, Permana PA, Yang X *et al*. A calpain-10 gene polymorphism is associated with reduced muscle mRNA levels and insulin resistance. *J Clin Invest* 2000; **106**(7):R69–73.
102. Sreenan SK, Zhou YP, Otani K *et al*. Calpains play a role in insulin secretion and action. *Diabetes* 2001; **50**(9):2013–20.
103. Stumvoll M, Fritsche A, Madaus A *et al*. Functional significance of the UCSNP-43 polymorphism in the CAPN10 gene for proinsulin processing and insulin secretion in nondiabetic Germans. *Diabetes* 2001; **50**(9):2161–3.
104. Hoffstedt J, Ryden M, Lofgren P *et al*. Polymorphism in the Calpain 10 gene influences glucose metabolism in human fat cells. *Diabetologia* 2002; **45**(2):276–82.
105. Hoffstedt J, Naslund E, Arner P. Calpain-10 gene polymorphism is associated with reduced beta(3)-adrenoceptor function in human fat cells. *J Clin Endocrinol Metab* 2002; **87**(7):3362–7.
106. Elbein SC, Hoffman MD, Teng K *et al*. A genome-wide search for type 2 diabetes susceptibility genes in Utah Caucasians. *Diabetes* 1999; **48**(5):1175–82.
107. Lynn S, Evans JC, White C *et al*. Variation in the calpain-10 gene affects blood glucose levels in the British population. *Diabetes* 2002; **51**(1):247–50.
108. Shore AC, Evans JC, Frayling TM *et al*. Association of calpain 10 and microvascular function. *Diabetologia* 2002; **45**(6):899–904.
109. Daimon M, Oizumi T, Saitoh T *et al*. Calpain 10 gene polymorphisms are related, not to type 2 diabetes, but to increased serum cholesterol in Japanese. *Diabetes Res Clin Pract* 2002; **56**(2):147–52.
110. Ehrmann DA, Schwarz PE, Hara M *et al*. Relationship of calpain-10 genotype to phenotypic features of polycystic ovary syndrome. *J Clin Endocrinol Metab* 2002; **87**(4):1669–73.
111. Haddad L, Evans JC, Gharani N *et al*. Variation within the type 2 diabetes susceptibility gene calpain-10 and polycystic ovary syndrome. *J Clin Endocrinol Metab* 2002; **87**(6):2606–10.
112. Huang Y, Wang KK. The calpain family and human disease. *Trends Mol Med* 2001; **7**(8):355–62.
113. Walder K, McMillan J, Lapsys N *et al*. Calpain 3 gene expression in skeletal muscle is associated with body fat content and measures of insulin resistance. *Int J Obes Relat Metab Disord* 2002; **26**(4):442–9.

114. Mahtani MM, Widen E, Lehto M *et al*. Mapping of a gene for type 2 diabetes associated with an insulin secretion defect by a genome scan in Finnish families. *Nat Genet* 1996; **14**(1):90–4.
115. Shaw JT, Lovelock PK, Kesting JB *et al*. Novel susceptibility gene for late-onset NIDDM is localized to human chromosome 12q. *Diabetes* 1998; **47**(11):1793–6.
116. Bektas A, Suprenant ME, Wogan LT *et al*. Evidence of a novel type 2 diabetes locus 50 cM centromeric to NIDDM2 on chromosome 12q. *Diabetes* 1999; **48**(11):2246–51.
117. Bektas A, Hughes JN, Warram JH *et al*. Type 2 diabetes locus on 12q15. Further mapping and mutation screening of two candidate genes. *Diabetes* 2001; **50**(1):204–8.
118. Duggirala R, Blangero J, Almasy L *et al*. Linkage of type 2 diabetes mellitus and of age at onset to a genetic location on chromosome 10q in Mexican Americans. *Am J Hum Genet* 1999; **64**(4):1127–40.
119. Mitchell BD, Cole SA, Hsueh WC *et al*. Linkage of serum insulin concentrations to chromosome 3p in Mexican Americans. *Diabetes* 2000; **49**(3):513–16.
120. Hanson RL, Ehm MG, Pettitt DJ *et al*. An autosomal genomic scan for loci linked to type II diabetes mellitus and body-mass index in Pima Indians. *Am J Hum Genet* 1998; **63**(4):1130–8.
121. Pratley RE, Thompson DB, Prochazka M *et al*. An autosomal genomic scan for loci linked to prediabetic phenotypes in Pima Indians. *J Clin Invest* 1998; **101**(8):1757–64.
122. Ghosh S, Watanabe RM, Valle TT *et al*. The Finland–United States investigation of non-insulin-dependent diabetes mellitus genetics (FUSION) study. I. An autosomal genome scan for genes that predispose to type 2 diabetes. *Am J Hum Genet* 2000; **67**(5):1174–85.
123. Ghosh S, Watanabe RM, Hauser ER *et al*. Type 2 diabetes: evidence for linkage on chromosome 20 in 716 Finnish affected sib pairs. *Proc Natl Acad Sci USA* 1999; **96**(5):2198–203.
124. Watanabe RM, Ghosh S, Langefeld CD *et al*. The Finland–United States investigation of non-insulin-dependent diabetes mellitus genetics (FUSION) study. II. An autosomal genome scan for diabetes-related quantitative-trait loci. *Am J Hum Genet* 2000; **67**(5):1186–200.
125. Vionnet N, Hani El-H, Dupont S *et al*. Genomewide search for type 2 diabetes-susceptibility genes in French whites: evidence for a novel susceptibility locus for early-onset diabetes on chromosome 3q27-qter and independent replication of a type 2-diabetes locus on chromosome 1q21–q24. *Am J Hum Genet* 2000; **67**(6):1470–80.
126. Ehm MG, Karnoub MC, Sakul H *et al*. Genome wide search for type 2 diabetes susceptibility genes in four American populations. *Am J Hum Genet* 2000; **66**(6):1871–81.
127. Permutt MA, Wasson JC, Suarez BK *et al*. A genome scan for type 2 diabetes susceptibility loci in a genetically isolated population. *Diabetes* 2001; **50**(3):681–5.
128. Meigs JB, Panhuysen CI, Myers RH *et al*. A genome-wide scan for loci linked to plasma levels of glucose and HbA(1c) in a community-based sample of

Caucasian pedigrees: The Framingham Offspring Study. *Diabetes* 2002; 51(3):833–40.

129. Mori Y, Otabe S, Dina C *et al.* Genome-wide search for type 2 diabetes in Japanese affected sib-pairs confirms susceptibility genes on 3q, 15q, and 20q and identifies two new candidate Loci on 7p and 11p. *Diabetes* 2002; 51(4):1247–55.

130. Stern MP. The search for type 2 diabetes susceptibility genes using whole-genome scans: an epidemiologist's perspective. *Diabetes Metab Res Rev* 2002; 18(2):106–13.

131. Fajans SS. Scope and heterogeneous nature of MODY. *Diabetes Care* 1990; 13:49-64.

132. Winter WE, Nakamura M, House DV. Monogenic diabetes mellitus in youth: The MODY syndromes. *Endocrinol Metabol Cl N Am* 1999; 28(4):765–85.

133. Winter WE, Maclaren NK, Riley WJ *et al.* Maturity-onset diabetes of youth in black Americans. *N Engl J Med* 1987; 316(6):285–91.

134. Weir GC, Sharma A, Zangen DH, Bonner-Weir S. Transcription factor abnormalities as a cause of beta cell dysfunction in diabetes: a hypothesis. *Acta Diabetol* 1997; 34(3):177–84.

135. Fajans SS, Bell GI, Polonsky KS. Molecular mechanisms and clinical pathophysiology of maturity-onset diabetes of the young. *N Engl J Med* 2001; 342:971–80.

136. Sander M, German MS. The beta cell transcription factors and development of the pancreas. *J Mol Med* 1997; 75(5):327–40.

137. Habener JF, Stoffers DA. A newly discovered role of transcription factors involved in pancreas development and the pathogenesis of diabetes mellitus. *Proc Ass Am Phys* 1998; 110(1):12–21.

138. Hattersley AT. Maturity-onset diabetes of the young: clinical heterogeneity explained by genetic heterogeneity. *Diabet Med* 1998; 15(1):15–24.

139. Hattersley AT. Diagnosis of maturity-onset diabetes of the young in the pediatric diabetes clinic. *J Pediatr Endocrinol Metab* 2000; 13(suppl 6): 1411–17.

140. Barrio R, Bellanne-Chantelot C, Moreno JC *et al.* Nine novel mutations in maturity-onset diabetes of the young (MODY) candidate genes in 22 Spanish families. *J Clin Endocrinol Metab* 2002; 87(6):2532–9.

141. Bell GI, Xiang KS, Newman MV, Wu SH *et al.* Gene for non-insulin-dependent diabetes mellitus (maturity-onset diabetes of the young subtype) is linked to DNA polymorphism on human chromosome 20q. *Proc Natl Acad Sci USA* 1991; 88(4):1484–8.

142. Yamagata K, Furuta H, Oda N *et al.* Mutations in the hepatocyte nuclear factor-4alpha gene in maturity-onset diabetes of the young (MODY1). *Nature* 1996; 384(6608):458–60.

143. Herman WH, Fajans SS, Ortiz FJ *et al.* Abnormal insulin secretion, not insulin resistance, is the genetic or primary defect of MODY in the RW pedigree. *Diabetes* 1994; 43(1):40–6.

144. Byrne MM, Sturis J, Fajans SS *et al.* Altered insulin secretory responses to glucose in subjects with a mutation in the MODY1 gene on chromosome 20. *Diabetes* 1995; 44(6):699–704.

145. Herman WH, Fajans SS, Smith MJ *et al.* Diminished insulin and glucagon secretory responses to arginine in nondiabetic subjects with a mutation in the hepatocyte nuclear factor-4alpha/MODY1 gene. *Diabetes* 1997; **46**(11): 1749–54.

146. Navas MA, Munoz-Elias EJ, Kim J *et al.* Functional characterization of the MODY1 gene mutations HNF4(R127W), HNF4(V255M), and HNF4(E276Q). *Diabetes* 1999; **48**(7):1459–65.

147. Suaud L, Hemimou Y, Formstecher P, Laine B. Functional study of the E276Q mutant hepatocyte nuclear factor-4alpha found in type 1 maturity-onset diabetes of the young: impaired synergy with chicken ovalbumin upstream promoter transcription factor II on the hepatocyte nuclear factor-1 promoter. *Diabetes* 1999; **48**(5):1162–7.

148. Yang Q, Yamagata K, Yamamoto K *et al.* R127W-HNF-4alpha is a loss of function mutation but not a rare polymorphism and causes type II diabetes in a Japanese family with MODY1. *Diabetologia* 2000; **43**(4):520–4.

149. Moller AM, Urhammer SA, Dalgaard LT *et al.* Studies of the genetic variability of the coding region of the hepatocyte nuclear factor-4alpha in Caucasians with maturity onset NIDDM. *Diabetologia* 1997; **40**(8): 980–3.

150. Yki-Jarvinen H. MODY genes and mutations in hepatocyte nuclear factors. *Lancet* 1997; **349**(9051):516–17.

151. Froguel P, Zouali H, Vionnet N *et al.* Familial hyperglycemia due to mutations in glucokinase. Definition of a subtype of diabetes mellitus. *N Engl J Med* 1993; **328**(10):697–702.

152. Froguel P, Vaxillaire M, Sun F *et al.* Close linkage of glucokinase locus on chromosome 7p to early-onset non-insulin-dependent diabetes mellitus. *Nature* 1992; **356**(6365):162–4.

153. Vionnet N, Stoffel M, Takeda J *et al.* Nonsense mutation in the glucokinase gene causes early-onset non-insulin-dependent diabetes mellitus. *Nature* 1992; **356**(6371):721–2.

154. Bell GI, Pilkis SJ, Weber IT, Polonsky KS. Glucokinase mutations, insulin secretion, and diabetes mellitus. *Annu Rev Physiol* 1996; **58**:171–86.

155. Hattersley AT, Beards F, Ballantyne E *et al.* Mutations in the glucokinase gene of the fetus result in reduced birth weight. *Nat Genet* 1998; **19**(3):268–70.

156. Polonsky KS. Lilly Lecture 1994. The beta-cell in diabetes: from molecular genetics to clinical research. *Diabetes* 1995; **44**(6):705–17.

157. Velho G, Blanche H, Vaxillaire M *et al.* Identification of 14 new glucokinase mutations and description of the clinical profile of 42 MODY-2 families. *Diabetologia* 1997; **40**(2):217–24.

158. Njolstad PR, Sovik O, Cuesta-Munoz A *et al.* Neonatal diabetes mellitus due to complete glucokinase deficiency. *N Engl J Med* 2001; **344**(21):1588–92.

159. Stoffel M, Bell KL, Blackburn CL *et al.* Identification of glucokinase mutations in subjects with gestational diabetes mellitus. *Diabetes* 1993; **42**(6): 937–40.

160. Chiu KC, Go RC, Aoki M *et al.* Glucokinase gene in gestational diabetes mellitus: population association study and molecular scanning. *Diabetologia* 1994; **37**(1):104–10.

161. Ellard S, Beards F, Allen LI *et al.* A high prevalence of glucokinase mutations in gestational diabetic subjects selected by clinical criteria. *Diabetologia* 2000; **43**(2):250–3.

162. Hattersley AT, Saker PJ, Cook JT *et al.* Microsatellite polymorphisms at the glucokinase locus: a population association study in Caucasian type 2 diabetic subjects. *Diabet Med* 1993; **10**(8):694–8.

163. Glaser B, Kesavan P, Heyman M *et al.* Familial hyperinsulinism caused by an activating glucokinase mutation. *N Engl J Med* 1998; **338**(4):226–30.

164. Christesen HB, Jacobsen BB, Odili S *et al.* The second activating glucokinase mutation (A456V): implications for glucose homeostasis and diabetes therapy. *Diabetes* 2002; **51**(4):1240–6.

165. Frayling TM, Bulamn MP, Ellard S *et al.* Mutations in the hepatocyte nuclear factor-1alpha gene are a common cause of maturity-onset diabetes of the young in the U.K. *Diabetes* 1997; **46**(4):720–5.

166. Gragnoli C, Lindner T, Cockburn BN *et al.* Maturity-onset diabetes of the young due to a mutation in the hepatocyte nuclear factor-4 alpha binding site in the promoter of the hepatocyte nuclear factor-1 alpha gene. *Diabetes* 1997; **46**(10):1648–51.

167. Lehto M, Tuomi T, Mahtani MM *et al.* Characterization of the MODY3 phenotype. Early-onset diabetes caused by an insulin secretion defect. *J Clin Invest* 1997; **99**(4):582–91.

168. Byrne MM, Sturis J, Menzel S *et al.* Altered insulin secretory responses to glucose in diabetic and nondiabetic subjects with mutations in the diabetes susceptibility gene MODY3 on chromosome 12. *Diabetes* 1996; **45**(11):1503–10.

169. Pearson ER, Liddell WG, Shepherd M *et al.* Sensitivity to sulphonylureas in patients with hepatocyte nuclear factor-1alpha gene mutations: evidence for pharmacogenetics in diabetes. *Diabet Med* 2000; **17**(7):543–5.

170. Ellard S. Hepatocyte nuclear factor 1 alpha (HNF-1 alpha) mutations in maturity-onset diabetes of the young. *Hum Mutat* 2000; **16**(5):377–85.

171. Stoffers DA, Zinkin NT, Stanojevic V *et al.* Pancreatic agenesis attributable to a single nucleotide deletion in the human IPF1 gene coding sequence. *Nat Gen* 1997; **15**:106–10.

172. Macfarlane WM, Frayling TM, Ellard S *et al.* Missense mutations in the insulin promoter factor-1 gene predispose to type 2 diabetes. *J Clin Invest* 1999; **104**(9):R33–9.

173. Clocquet AR, Egan JM, Stoffers DA *et al.* Impaired insulin secretion and increased insulin sensitivity in familial maturity-onset diabetes of the young 4 (insulin promoter factor 1 gene). *Diabetes* 2000; **49**(11):1856–64.

174. Hani EH, Stoffers DA, Chevre JC *et al.* Defective mutations in the insulin promoter factor-1 (IPF-1) gene in late-onset type 2 diabetes mellitus. *J Clin Invest* 1999; **104**(9):R41–8.

175. Weng J, Macfarlane WM, Lehto M *et al.* Functional consequences of mutations in the MODY4 gene (IPF1) and coexistence with MODY3 mutations. *Diabetologia* 2001; **44**(2):249–58.

176. Hansen L, Urioste S, Petersen HV *et al.* Missense mutations in the human insulin promoter factor-1 gene and their relation to maturity-onset diabetes of the young and late-onset type 2 diabetes mellitus in caucasians. *J Clin Endocrinol Metab* 2000; **85**(3):1323–6.

177. Reis AF, Ye WZ, Dubois-Laforgue D *et al*. Mutations in the insulin promoter factor-1 gene in late-onset type 2 diabetes mellitus. *Eur J Endocrinol* 2000; **143**(4):511–13.

178. Horikawa Y, Iwasaki N, Hara M *et al*. Mutation in hepatocyte nuclear factor-1 beta gene (TCF2) associated with MODY. *Nat Genet* 1997; **17**(4):384–5.

179. Lindner TH, Njolstad PR, Horikawa Y *et al*. A novel syndrome of diabetes mellitus, renal dysfunction and genital malformation associated with a partial deletion of the pseudo-POU domain of hepatocyte nuclear factor-1 beta. *Hum Mol Genet* 1999; **8**(11):2001–8.

180. Bingham C, Ellard S, Allen L *et al*. Abnormal nephron development associated with a frameshift mutation in the transcription factor hepatocyte nuclear factor-1 beta. *Kidney Int* 2000; **57**(3):898–907.

181. Nishigori H, Yamada S, Kohama T *et al*. Frameshift mutation, A263fsinsGG, in the hepatocyte nuclear factor-1beta gene associated with diabetes and renal dysfunction. *Diabetes* 1998; **47**(8):1354–5.

182. Beards F, Frayling T, Bulman M *et al*. Mutations in hepatocyte nuclear factor 1 beta are not a common cause of maturity-onset diabetes of the young in the U.K. *Diabetes* 1998; **47**(7):1152–4.

183. Furuta H, Furuta M, Sanke T *et al*. Nonsense and missense mutations in the human hepatocyte nuclear factor -1 beta gene (TCF2) and their relation to type 2 diabetes in Japanese. *J Clin Endocrinol Metab* 2002; **87**(8):3859–63.

184. Kristinsson SY, Thorolfsdottir ET, Talseth B *et al*. MODY in Iceland is associated with mutations in HNF-1alpha and a novel mutation in NeuroD1. *Diabetologia* 2001; **44**(11):2098–101.

185. Malecki MT, Jhala US, Antonellis A *et al*. Mutations in NEUROD1 are associated with the development of type 2 diabetes mellitus. *Nat Genet* 1999; **23**(3):323–8.

186. Furuta H, Horikawa Y, Iwasaki N *et al*. Beta-cell transcription factors and diabetes: mutations in the coding region of the BETA2/NeuroD1 (NEUROD1) and Nkx2.2 (NKX2B) genes are not associated with maturity-onset diabetes of the young in Japanese. *Diabetes* 1998; **47**(8):1356–8.

187. Naya FJ, Huang HP, Qiu Y *et al*. Diabetes, defective pancreatic morphogenesis, and abnormal enteroendocrine differentiation in BETA2/neuroD-deficient mice. *Genes Dev* 1997; **11**(18):2323–34.

188. Froguel P, Velho G. Molecular genetics of maturity-onset diabetes of the young. *Trends Endocrinol Metab* 1999; **10**(4):142–6.

189. Doria A, Yang Y, Malecki M *et al*. Phenotypic characteristics of early-onset autosomal-dominant type 2 diabetes unlinked to known maturity-onset diabetes of the young (MODY) genes. *Diabetes Care* 1999; **22**(2):253–61.

190. Dussoix P, Vaxillaire M, Iynedjian PB *et al*. Diagnostic heterogeneity of diabetes in lean young adults: classification based on immunological and genetic parameters. *Diabetes* 1997; **46**(4):622–31.

191. Yu L, Wei Q, Jin L *et al*. Genetic variation in the hepatocyte nuclear factor (HNF)-3alpha gene does not contribute to maturity-onset diabetes of the young in Japanese. *Horm Metab Res* 2001; **33**(3):163–6.

192. Yamada S, Zhu Q, Aihara Y *et al*. Cloning of cDNA and the gene encoding human hepatocyte nuclear factor (HNF)-3 beta and mutation screening in Japanese subjects with maturity-onset diabetes of the young. *Diabetologia* 2000; **43**(1):121–4.

193. Hinokio Y, Horikawa Y, Furuta H *et al*. Beta-cell transcription factors and diabetes: no evidence for diabetes-associated mutations in the hepatocyte nuclear factor-3beta gene (HNF3B) in Japanese patients with maturity-onset diabetes of the young. *Diabetes* 2000; **49**(2):302–5.

194. Abderrahmani A, Chevre JC, Otabe S *et al*. Genetic variation in the hepatocyte nuclear factor-3beta gene (HNF3B) does contribute to maturity-onset diabetes of the young in French Caucasians. *Diabetes* 2000; **49**(2):306–8.

195. Hara M, Wang X, Paz VP *et al*. No diabetes-associated mutations in the coding region of the hepatocyte nuclear factor-4gamma gene (HNF4G) in Japanese patients with MODY. *Diabetologia* 2000; **43**(8):1064–9.

196. Plengvidhya N, Antonellis A, Wogan LT *et al*. Hepatocyte nuclear factor-4gamma: cDNA sequence, gene organization, and mutation screening in early-onset autosomal-dominant type 2 diabetes. *Diabetes* 1999; **48**(10): 2099–102.

197. Zhu Q, Yamagata K, Tsukahara Y *et al*. Mutation screening of the hepatocyte nuclear factor (HNF)-6 gene in Japanese subjects with diabetes mellitus. *Diabetes Res Clin Pract* 2001; **52**(3):171–4.

198. Horikawa Y, Horikawa Y, Cox NJ *et al*. Beta-cell transcription factors and diabetes: no evidence for diabetes-associated mutations in the gene encoding the basic helix–loop–helix transcription factor neurogenic differentiation 4 (NEUROD4) in Japanese patients with MODY. *Diabetes* 2000; **49**(11):1955–7.

199. del Bosque-Plata L, Lin J, Horikawa Y *et al*. Mutations in the coding region of the neurogenin 3 gene (NEUROG3) are not a common cause of maturity-onset diabetes of the young in Japanese subjects. *Diabetes* 2001; **50**(3):694–6.

200. Jensen JN, Hansen L, Ekstrom CT *et al*. Polymorphisms in the neurogenin 3 gene (NEUROG) and their relation to altered insulin secretion and diabetes in the Danish Caucasian population. *Diabetologia* 2001; **44**(1): 123–6.

201. Schwartz M, Vissing J. Paternal inheritance of mitochondrial DNA. *N Engl J Med* 2002; **347**(8):576–8.

202. Howell N. Mitochondrial gene mutations and human disease: a prolegomenon. *Am J Hum Genet* 1994; **55**:219–24.

203. Johns DR. Mitochondrial DNA and disease. *N Engl J Med* 1995; **333**:638–44.

204. Anderson S, Bankier AT, Barrell BG *et al*. Sequence and organization of the human mitochondrial genome. *Nature* 1981; **290**(5806):457–65.

205. Maechler P, Wollheim CB. Mitochondrial function in normal and diabetic beta-cells. *Nature* 2001; **414**(6865):807–12.

206. Maassen JA, Janssen GM, Lemkes HH. Mitochondrial diabetes mellitus. *J Endocrinol Invest* 2002; **25**(5):477–84.

207. Singhal N, Gupta BS, Saigal R *et al*. Mitochondrial diseases: an overview of genetics, pathogenesis, clinical features and an approach to diagnosis and treatment. *J Postgrad Med* 2000; **46**(3):224–30.

208. van den Ouweland JM, Lemkes HH, Ruitenbeek W *et al*. Mutation in mitochondrial tRNA(Leu)(UUR) gene in a large pedigree with maternally transmitted type II diabetes mellitus and deafness. *Nat Genet* 1992; **1**(5):368–71.

209. Lee WJ, Lee HW, Palmer JP *et al*. Islet cell autoimmunity and mitochondrial DNA mutation in Korean subjects with typical and atypical type I diabetes. *Diabetologia* 2001; **44**(12):2187–91.

210. Oka Y, Katagiri H, Yazaki Y *et al.* Mitochondrial gene mutation in islet-cell-antibody-positive patients who were initially non-insulin-dependent diabetics. *Lancet* 1993; **342**(8870):527–8.
211. Kadowaki T, Kadowaki H, Mori Y *et al.* A subtype of diabetes mellitus associated with a mutation of mitochondrial DNA. *N Engl J Med* 1994; **330**(14):962–8.
212. Reardon W, Ross RJ, Sweeney MG *et al.* Diabetes mellitus associated with a pathogenic point mutation in mitochondrial DNA. *Lancet* 1992; **340**(8832):1376–9.
213. Choo-Kang AT, Lynn S, Taylor GA *et al.* Defining the importance of mitochondrial gene defects in maternally inherited diabetes by sequencing the entire mitochondrial genome. *Diabetes* 2002; **51**(7):2317–20.
214. Thakker RV. Multiple endocrine neoplasia. *Horm Res* 2001; **56**(suppl 1): 67–72.
215. Roy J, Pompilio M, Samama G. Pancreatic somatostatinoma and MEN 1. Apropos of a case. Review of the literature. *Ann Endocrinol (Paris)* 1996; **57**(1):71–6.
216. Koch CA, Vortmeyer AO, Huang SC *et al.* Genetic aspects of pheochromocytoma. *Endocr Regul* 2001; **35**(1):43–52.
217. Flier JS, Kahn CR, Roth J. Receptors, antireceptor antibodies and mechanisms of insulin resistance. *N Engl J Med* 1979; **300**(8):413–19.
218. Taylor SI, Kadowaki T, Kadowaki H *et al.* Mutations in insulin-receptor gene in insulin-resistant patients. *Diabetes Care* 1990; **13**(3):257–79.
219. Longo N, Wang Y, Pasquali M. Progressive decline in insulin levels in Rabson–Mendenhall syndrome. *J Clin Endocrinol Metab* 1999; **84**(8): 2623–9.
220. Yung B, Noormohamed FH, Kemp M *et al.* Cystic fibrosis-related diabetes: the role of peripheral insulin resistance and beta-cell dysfunction. *Diabet Med* 2002; **19**(3):221–6.
221. Khanim F, Kirk J, Latif F, Barrett TG. WFS1/wolframin mutations, Wolfram syndrome, and associated diseases. *Hum Mutat* 2001; **17**(5):357–67.
222. Inoue H, Tanizawa Y, Wasson J *et al.* A gene encoding a transmembrane protein is mutated in patients with diabetes mellitus and optic atrophy (Wolfram syndrome). *Nat Genet* 1998; **20**(2):143–8.
223. Takeda K, Inoue H, Tanizawa Y *et al.* WFS1 (Wolfram syndrome 1) gene product: predominant subcellular localization to endoplasmic reticulum in cultured cells and neuronal expression in rat brain. *Hum Mol Genet* 2001; **10**(5):477–84.
224. Cryns K, Pfister M, Pennings RJ *et al.* Mutations in the WFS1 gene that cause low-frequency sensorineural hearing loss are small non-inactivating mutations. *Hum Genet* 2002; **110**(5):389–94.
225. Minton JA, Hattersley AT, Owen K *et al.* Association studies of genetic variation in the WFS1 gene and type 2 diabetes in U.K. populations. *Diabetes* 2002; **51**(4):1287–90.
226. Yamada K, Ikegami H, Yoneda H *et al.* All patients with Werner's syndrome are insulin resistant, but only those who also have impaired insulin secretion develop overt diabetes. *Diabetes Care* 1999; **22**(12):2094–5.
227. Furuichi Y. Premature aging and predisposition to cancers caused by mutations in RecQ family helicases. *Ann NY Acad Sci* 2001; **928**:121–31.

228. Green JS, Parfrey PS, Harnett JD *et al*. The cardinal manifestations of Bardet–Biedl syndrome, a form of Laurence–Moon–Biedl syndrome. *N Engl J Med* 1989; **321**(15):1002–9.
229. Mykytyn K, Nishimura DY, Searby CC *et al*. Identification of the gene (BBS1) most commonly involved in Bardet–Biedl syndrome, a complex human obesity syndrome. *Nat Genet* 2002; **31**(4):435–8.
230. Kumar PG, Laloraya M, She JX. Population genetics and functions of the autoimmune regulator (AIRE). *Endocrinol Metab Clin North Am* 2002; **31**(2):321–38.
231. Brandhagen DJ, Fairbanks VF, Batts KP, Thibodeau SN. Update on hereditary hemochromatosis and the HFE gene. *Mayo Clin Proc* 1999; **74**(9): 917–21.
232. Haddy TB, Castro OL, Rana SR. Hereditary hemochromatosis in children, adolescents, and young adults. *Am J Pediatr Hematol Oncol* 1988; **10**(1): 23–34.
233. Schuster DP, Osei K, Zipf WB. Characterization of alterations in glucose and insulin metabolism in Prader–Willi subjects. *Metabolism* 1996; **45**(12): 1514–20.
234. Zipf WB. Glucose homeostasis in Prader–Willi syndrome and potential implications of growth hormone therapy. *Acta Paediatr Suppl* 1999; **88**(433): 115–17.
235. Das S, Lese CM, Song M *et al*. Partial paternal uniparental disomy of chromosome 6 in an infant with neonatal diabetes, macroglossia, and craniofacial abnormalities. *Am J Hum Genet* 2000; **67**(6):1586–91.
236. Garg A. Lipodystrophies. *Am J Med* 2000; **108**(2):143–52.
237. Agarwal AK, Arioglu E, De Almeida S *et al*. AGPAT2 is mutated in congenital generalized lipodystrophy linked to chromosome 9q34. *Nat Genet* 2002; **31**(1):21–3.
238. Magre J, Delepine M, Khallouf E *et al*. Identification of the gene altered in Berardinelli–Seip congenital lipodystrophy on chromosome 11q13. *Nat Genet* 2001; **28**(4):365–70.
239. Cao H, Hegele RA. Nuclear lamin A/C R482Q mutation in Canadian kindreds with Dunnigan-type familial partial lipodystrophy. *Hum Mol Genet* 2000; **9**(1):109–12.
240. Agarwal AK, Garg A. A novel heterozygous mutation in peroxisome proliferator-activated receptor-gamma gene in a patient with familial partial lipodystrophy. *J Clin Endocrinol Metab* 2002; **87**(1):408–11.
241. Matyka KA, Beards F, Appleton M *et al*. Genetic testing for maturity onset diabetes of the young in childhood hyperglycaemia. *Arch Dis Child* 1998; **78**(6):552–4.
242. Guazzarotti L, Bartolotta E, Chiarelli F. Maturity-onset diabetes of the young (MODY): a new challenge for pediatric diabetologists. *J Pediatr Endocrinol Metab* 1999; **12**(4):487–97.

Index

Page numbers in *italics* indicate figures or tables.